# Breast and Gynecological Cancers - New Perspectives and Applications in Their Treatment

*Edited by Michael Friedrich*

Published in London, United Kingdom

Breast and Gynecological Cancers - New Perspectives and Applications in Their Treatment
http://dx.doi.org/10.5772/intechopen.1003588
Edited by Michael Friedrich

Contributors
Abhiram Kumar, Abubakr Mohamed Ali Nasr, Chhavi Dhiman, Hoosdally Shakeel, Kumar Pranav Narayan, Maede Makhtoomi, Mani Sharma, Marzieh Mahmoodi, Masoud Amini Kahrizsangi, Mehran Nouri, Merve Konal, Mohini Rawat, Nemala Siva Kumar, Pegah Hadi Sichani, Piyush Khandelia, Rama Satya Sri Kotipalli, Tamara Kalir, Zainab Shateri



First published in London, United Kingdom, 2025 by IntechOpen
IntechOpen is the global imprint of INTECHOPEN LIMITED, registered in England and Wales, registration number: 11086078, 167-169 Great Portland Street, London, W1W 5PF, United Kingdom

For EU product safety concerns: IN TECH d.o.o., Prolaz Marije Krucifikse Kozulić 3, 51000 Rijeka, Croatia, info@intechopen.com or visit our website at intechopen.com.

British Library Cataloguing-in-Publication Data
A catalogue record for this book is available from the British Library

Breast and Gynecological Cancers - New Perspectives and Applications in Their Treatment
Edited by Michael Friedrich
p. cm.

This title is part of the Oncology Book Series, Volume 3
Series Editor: Thomas J. FitzGerald

Print ISBN 978-1-83634-005-8
Online ISBN 978-1-83634-004-1
eBook (PDF) ISBN 978-1-83634-006-5
ISSN 3049-8864

If disposing of this product, please recycle the paper responsibly.

# IntechOpen Book Series
# Oncology
## Volume 3

## Aims and Scope of the Series

The field of oncology has undergone extraordinary change and progress over the past several decades. Today, information is evolving at a rapid rate, with standards of management far different than standards of care applied during the training of most practicing oncologists. Oncology practitioners in all disciplines must remain current to optimize patient care. Basic and translational science remain critical in developing process improvements for patient care. The closer we understand the mechanism, the more we can improve targeted therapies and apply them to patient care. The pace of information is moving faster than at any previous time in history, and all oncology disciplines must remain current to provide excellent service to patients. The modern oncologist must be fluent in using big data and the volume of information generated in clinical trials. As we move closer to personalized patient care based on genomics and molecular biomarkers, the modern oncologist has to be nimble in assessing all available information and how this would be applied to each patient, balanced by the clinical status and medical co-morbidities of each patient. Targeted therapies can bring new and different sequelae, and oncology teams need to remain fluent in managing the consequences of therapy and primary management. In this book series, we will present how modern care has progressed in multiple disease areas and how modern oncology teams need to adapt in order to manage the cancer patients of today successfully. Surgery, radiation therapy, and medical oncology are practiced today with the support of exceptional modern technology, and in this series, we will review how these improvements are applied to each disease site to maintain excellence in patient care.

# Meet the Series Editor

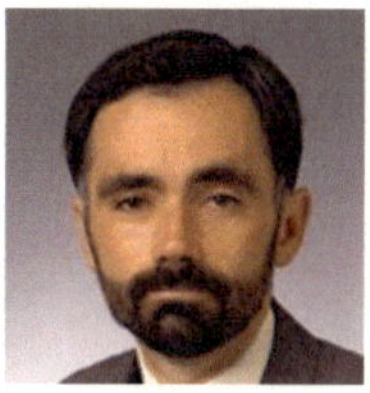

Dr. FitzGerald is the professor and chair of the Department of Radiation Oncology at UMass Chan Medical School in the USA. He serves as one of the principal investigators of the Imaging and Radiation Oncology Core (IROC) service for the National Cancer Institute clinical trials program and is directly involved in the quality assurance of clinical trials in the National Clinical Trials Network (NCTN). Dr. Fitzgerald manages NCTN clinical trials with a real-time pre-therapy review of imaging and radiation therapy treatment objects to ensure the care plan complies with study objectives and the patient stage has been assigned to the correct study. His basic science interest is in hematopoietic stem cell biology and cellular adhesion molecules as they pertain to therapeutic resistance and mitigation of injury from therapy.

# Meet the Volume Editor

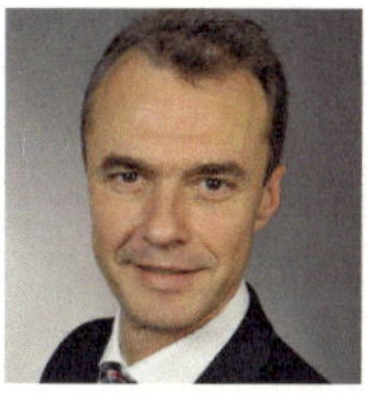

Michael Friedrich is a senior gynecological oncologist and oncological surgeon at Helios Klinikum Krefeld, Germany, and specializes in treating women with breast cancer and gynecological malignancies. He is a certified breast surgeon and has an academic appointment as an associate professor at the University of Schleswig-Holstein, Germany. He has received several awards for his scientific work, which focuses on vitamin D metabolism in gynecologic malignancies and the interaction of DNA-mismatch repair and resistance to chemotherapy. Further research interests are interstitial brachytherapy for recurrences of cervical cancer, the use of innovative therapies in gynecological malignancies, the sentinel lymph node technique in gynecological malignancies, especially in vulvar cancer, and the use of intraoperative intraperitoneal chemotherapy (HIPEC) in ovarian cancer. Dr. Friedrich is a member of several prestigious editorial and scientific boards and a member of Germany's committees for S3 guidelines for cervical, endometrial, vulvar, and breast cancer. He is also a member of the Ethics Committee of the Nordrhein-Westfalen Medical Chamber, the board of directors of the BLFG (Bundesarbeitsgemeinschaft leitender Frauenärzte), the board of the German Society for Gynecology, where he is responsible for developing the continuous medical education curriculum in gynecology, and the Society of Pelvic Surgeons.

# Contents

# Preface

The management of gynecologic cancer has evolved tremendously in the last few years. This book will focus on individualized treatment strategies for different gynecologic malignancies.

*Breast and Gynecological Cancers – New Perspectives and Applications in Their Treatment* represents a review of interesting and clinically important advances in the tumor biology and treating breast and gynecologic malignancies. Major aspects of scientific progress in the treatment of gynecologic malignancies with regard to new knowledge due to advances in the understanding of tumor biology and innovative new medical treatment options are covered. An interesting collection of innovative aspects in the diagnosis and treatment of gynecological malignancies and opinions from specialists who are relevant to this field are brought together in this book.

Uterine leiomyosarcoma (ULMS) is an uncommon gynecological cancer, and treatments such as surgical debulking, chemotherapy, and radiotherapy have had limited results. Identifying small molecules could essentially be utilized for personalized treatment of leiomyosarcoma, especially with patients carrying the tp53 mutations. The first chapter of the book will focus on the concept of personalized tumor therapy for uterine leiomyosarcoma.

Ovarian cancer screening remains elusive despite tireless efforts. The challenges faced include the prevalence of ovarian cancer and its impact on the positive predictive value of screening tests. Effective screening is crucial, as this is the deadliest gynecological cancer and often presents at a late stage. The diversity of the targeted population, low and high risk, as well as the ambiguity in oncogenesis and shared origin by fallopian tubes and peritoneum, are genuine obstacles in unifying a screening program for the heterogeneous disease. The consensus does not recommend screening in low-risk populations. Evaluating available screening tests in multiple trials did not prove a reduction in mortality. There may be an increase in detection of early disease. However, the impact on mortality and quality of life is questionable. The second chapter will discuss these different aspects.

Endometrial cancer is the most common uterine malignancy in the U.S. and Europe and a significant cause of morbidity and mortality in these countries. While there was good agreement among pathologists in the diagnosis of low-grade (well and moderately differentiated) endometrial carcinomas, the same could not be said for all high-grade tumors. In 2013, a new, 4-tier molecular classification scheme for the pathologic diagnosis of endometrial cancer was proposed with ground-breaking implications, which will be evaluated in the third chapter.

Cervical cancer remains a significant health concern globally, particularly in low- and middle-income countries. Accurate staging of cervical cancer is critical as it directly influences treatment decisions and prognostic assessments. This chapter provides a comprehensive overview of the staging methodologies used in cervical cancer, highlighting the International Federation of Gynecology and Obstetrics (FIGO) and the Tumor, Node, Metastasis (TNM) staging systems. It delves into diagnostic methods, including clinical examination, advanced imaging techniques, and pathological evaluation, and discusses recent advancements such as molecular imaging, biomarkers, and artificial intelligence. The fourth chapter also explores the clinical implications of staging, including its role in treatment planning, prognostic evaluation, and follow-up care.

Breast cancer is the second most common cancer and one of the most common cancers in women worldwide. The risk factors of this cancer can be classified into two categories: non-modifiable and modifiable. It has been shown that modifiable lifestyle factors, such as diet, play an important role in cancer prevention. Recently, instead of using specific foods as indicators of dietary intake and nutritional status, component food group analysis has been used to determine dietary patterns. Although the findings are insufficient to evaluate the relationship between diet and breast cancer risk, a reduction in breast cancer risk has been reported following an increase in fruit and vegetable consumption. This is described in the fifth chapter.

Cancer stem cells are a crucial subpopulation in gynecological tumors, defined by their self-renewal, differentiation potential, and resistance to conventional therapies. These cells are central to tumor initiation, progression, metastasis, and recurrence, making them key targets for innovative therapeutic strategies. The last chapter will explore the molecular mechanisms that regulate cancer stem cells, focusing on signalling pathways such as Wnt, Notch, and Hedgehog, which are critical for cancer stem cell maintenance and survival. It will also examine emerging therapeutic approaches aimed at eradicating cancer stem cells, including pathway inhibitors, immune-based strategies, and combinatorial treatments. Further, this chapter delves into the challenges and future directions of translating cancer stem cell-targeted therapies into clinical practice.

**Michael Friedrich**
Department of Obstetrics and Gynecology,
Helios Hospital,
Krefeld, Germany

**Chapter 1**

# Computational Methods for Personalized Targeted Therapy in Uterine Leiomyosacoma

*Hoosdally Shakeel*


## Abstract

Uterine leiomyosarcoma (ULMS) is an uncommon gynecological cancer, and treatments such as surgical debulking, chemotherapy, and radiotherapy have had limited results. This investigation study is about a scenario of a 53- year-old woman, whereby conventional protocol through combining doxetatacel, gemcitabine, pazopanib, pemetrexed, and doxorubicin with surgery and radiation did not avoid metastasis, resulting in the death of the patient. A strategy of personalized tumor therapy was used. Through the recommendation of a ctdna (circulating tumor DNA) next-generation sequencing (NGS) using blood sample, the mutated tp53 c338y was identified. A built homology of the mutated TP 53 proteins with a drug library of 1133 FDA approved drugs can be used in repurposing as part of the therapy regimen. Virtual drug screening using molecular docking was performed with PyRx 0.8 and dockey software. The top 10 drugs were found to bind to the target genes. Three from the top 10 were further refined with AutoDock 4.2.6. The identification of small molecules could essentially be utilized for personalized leiomyosarcoma, specially with patients carrying the tp53 mutations. This concept of personalized tumor therapy could be effective not only for uterine leiomyosarcoma but for other tumors as well.


**Keywords:** repurposed drugs, virtual screening, homology model, uterine leiomyosarcoma, molecular docking, computer software, personalized tumor therapy, next generation sequencing (NGS)

## 1. Introduction

ULMS is a malignant mesenchymal form of neoplasm accounting for 10–20% of newly diagnosed sarcoma [1, 2]. ULMS have a poor prognosis and aggressive biological behavior with local and distant metastasis. Although most cases are sporadic, li Fraumeni syndrome is a risk factor [3]. Patients have a high risk of relapse, and 80% of relapse occurs within the first 2 years [4]. ULMS is a highly complex karyotype with genomic instability. Patients with disseminated ULMS are usually incurable with median survival of 1 year after development of distant metastasis [5].

Genomic molecular profiling of ULMS shows alterations and mutations or deletions in tumor suppressor genes TP53, RB, ATRX, and PTEN [6]. Omics findings have shown a high level of alternate lengthening of telemores and defects in Homologous

Recombination (HR) and DNA repair pathway [7, 8]. ULMS exhibits low tumor molecular burden (TMB) with 2–5 mutations per megabase. Genomic analysis has identified homologous recombination DNA repair pathway HRD [8–12]. Additional alternated genes identified are TP53, C-MYC/RET, CDK N2A/B, NF1, RB1, BRCA2, and FGFR.

The current treatments of ULMS involve surgical debulking, radiotherapy, and adjuvant chemotherapy. First-line settings with patients with advanced ULMS are treated with doxorubicin or gemcitabine combined with docetaxel [13]. ULMS appears to be sensitive to gemcitabine-docetaxel with a therapeutic rate of 35.8% and Median Progression Free Survival (PFS) of 4.4 months [13]. Conventional treatments including surgery radiation and combinational chemotherapy using doxetacel/gemcitabine, maid protocol, and premetrexed did not improve the patient condition and yielded no survival benefits [14]. Radiation destabilizes the DNA structure and triggers protein kinase pathways, which blocks cell cycle progression. Tp53 is the key effector in DNA damage-activated kinase pathways, and the key aim of Tp53 is to promote cellular apoptosis [15]. Hence, the need arose performing genomic profiling of a tumor before selecting cancer therapies.

Different recurrent alterations are observed in ULMS in different patients. Advanced genomic profiling is needed to identify oncogene drivers, and the need for personalized therapy for each patient is warranted. Many studies have shown that gene mutations cause uncontrolled cell growth and resistance to conventional antitumor treatment. Targeted oncology addresses this issue by using the genomic landscape of the tumor to find gene alterations where targeted therapies can be implemented. But there is scarcity of drugs to target these mutations. Targeted therapies have shown increased rate of survival compared to classical chemotherapy protocols [14]. We should also bear in mind that tumors have clonal and sub-clonal populations. The greater the degree of heterogeneity, the less effective response from chemotherapy.

Drug repurposing is an interesting concept that uses already FDA- approved drugs that were indicated for further diseases other than cancer [16]. These drugs have already passed safety and toxicity phases in clinical trials. This concept is interesting from both an economic and medical perspective as it takes around 15 years to bring a new drug on the marketplace with a huge amount of money being invested. Repurposed drugs should be encouraged in all cancer types. A classic example is metformin initially approved for diabetes has shown activity against gastrointestinal tumors [17].

The present investigation is about a 53 -year-old female patient suffering from ULMS. The clinical history of the condition was described, whereby genomic mutational landscape was established by NGS. The identification of mutations from NGS was mapped to conduct virtual screening using a database of 1123 FDA-approved drugs to devise new treatment strategies for this uncurable disease. The above strategy can be adopted in cases where personalized treatment of cancer patients runs out of treatment protocol.

## 2. Case presentation

A 53-year-old woman living in Mauritius was treated in a New Cancer Centre (NCC) established in Mauritius. She was initially diagnosed of ULMS in 2019 and suffered from stage 4 lung metastasis. In April 2019, a CT scan revealed a significant fibroid uterus, leading to a diagnosis of uterine leiomyosarcoma. Further in May 2019, a mass of 210 mm in maximum dimension was extended into the deep endocervix.

A complete hysterectomy was performed. Subsequently, she underwent treatment with six cycles of doxetacel and gemcitabine from June 2019 to November 2019. In January 2020, she underwent external radiotherapy specifically targeting the uterine area. The Position Emission Tomography (PET) scan result showed significant hypermetabolic activity in pelvic lymph nodes. Hypermetabolic nodules and mass lesions were noted in bilateral lungs, suggestive of metastasis. Fluorodeoxyglucose (FDG) uptake was seen in pleural-based and parenchymal soft tissue density mass lesions and nodules in bilateral lung parenchyma (largest in posterior and lateral basal segment of the left lower lobe measuring 8.6 x 5.8 cm) SUV value of 28. Further, in May 2022, a regimen of six cycles of docetaxel/gemcitabine was initiated. In December 2022, she began taking pazopanib tablets, a tyrosine kinase inhibitor. Despite the above regimen, in January 2024, cannonball lung metastases were seen by PET-CT scan of the thorax with bilateral pleural effusions and right pneumothorax. Diffusely scattered, heterogeneously enhancing lobulated lesions of varying sizes containing internal areas of necrosis were seen in all lobes of both lungs. In March 2024, her treating oncologist of NCC recommended the mesna, doxorubicin, ifosfamide, and dacarbazine (MAID) protocol and premetrexed. On 19-Mar-2024, an NGS analysis of blood CT DNA was performed to get a genomic profile of the tumor and any actionable genes for molecular targeted therapies.

## 2.1 Test conducted

### *2.1.1 DNA sequence variant*

The data from **Table 1**. was extracted from the Patient Report NGSS conducted at a local clinic in Mauritius (Clinic Wellkin - Mauritius)

## 2.2 Materials and methods

Based on **Table 1** and according to CLINVAR (https://www.ncbi.nlm.nih.gov/clinvar/), the main drivers' mutations are TP53C238Y and p. (Q331Hfs*6), which are highly pathogenic. Furthermore, the PDGFAR is a benign variant and will not be considered further for this study.

The tumor-suppressor protein TP53 has been involved in almost 60% of all human cancer cases. It is crucial to scrutinize the structure and purpose of TP53 and how it threatens cell reliability when mutations are formed [18]. On chromosome 17p 13.1, the TP53 gene consists of 393 AA. The sequence-specific DNA-binding domain (AAs 102–292) is the core part of TP53. In tumors, TP53 missense mutations are thought to be prevailing, specially influencing amino acids located near the DNA-binding surface of the gene. According to the International Agency for Research on Cancer (IARC) TP53 Mutation Database (28) lists, 95% of these oncogenic mutations are located in the DNA-binding domain (DBD). Mutated TP53 was found to be resistant to several conventional drugs that are used in therapy such as cisplatin, doxorubicin, cetuximab, and gemcitabine [19]. It is well known that stabilizing the destabilizing mutants of TP53 is a prospectus to treat tumors. Till now the TP53 has been undruggable, but a recent report by Pradhan et al. [20] has identified the S6-S7 pocket to be druggable.

## 2.3 Homology building model of the mutated TP53 c238 y

The main driver mutation for this patient was (TP53):c.713G > A (p.Cys238Tyr). There has been a change in the amino acid residue at position 238

| Gene | Amino acid change | Coding | Variant ID | Locus | Transcript | Variant effect |
|---|---|---|---|---|---|---|
| PDGFAR | p(S478P) | C.1432 T > C | | chr4:55139771 | NM_006206.6 | Missense |
| TP53 | p.(Q331Hfs*6) | c.992_993insT | | chr17:7576853 | NM_000546.6 | Frameshift insertion |
| TP53 | p. (C238Y) | c.713G > A | p.C238Y | chr17:757568 | NM_000546.6 | Missense |

**Table 1.**
*Relevant mutations in the ULMS patient.*

in TP53 whereby cysterine was replaced by tyrosine. The P53 c238y mutated gene 3D crystallographic structure has not yet been annotated in the Protein Drug Bank (PDB) database. Hence, the amino acid sequence of the mutated TP53, having accession number (P04637), was retrieved from the Uniprot database (https://www.uniprot.org/uniprotkb/P04637/entry#VAR_005967) in the FASTA format. The model was built using the Swiss model server (https://swissmodel.expasy.org/interactive) with a template of the new TP53 monomer structure PDB id (8F2I), as illustrated in **Figure 1**.

The model structure of the target protein was refined using the high-resolution protein structure refinement tool (ModRefiner) of the Zhang Lab online server (https://zhanggroup.org/ModRefiner/) and GalaxyRefine (https://galaxy.seoklab.org/). GalaxyRefine is a web server for protein structure prediction, refinement, and related methods.

### 2.4 Validation of the model

The model of c238y was validated by the SAVES server (https://saves.mbi.ucla.edu/). The tools of the SAVES server consist of the following: ERRAT, VERIFY3D, and PROCHECK resulted as follows. PROCHECK analysis delivered a Ramachandran plot for the given protein structures (Modeler-generated TP53 mutated c238y). The results of PROCHECK's Ramachandran plot for the given model are shown in **Figure 2**, and their data are tabulated in **Tables 2** and **3**.

The mutated model generated was superimposed on the TP53(PDB ID:8F2I) as per **Figure 3**. FATCAT is a server which is used for alignment of models. The RMSD value obtained upon alignment is 1.23 angstrom (Å), suggesting a very good model of the mutated TP53. A value between 0.5 < TM-score < 1.00 is considered very good. The TM score was 0.97248, and RMSD was 1.23 Å. In general, an RMSD value of less than 2 Å is considered a very good, validated model.

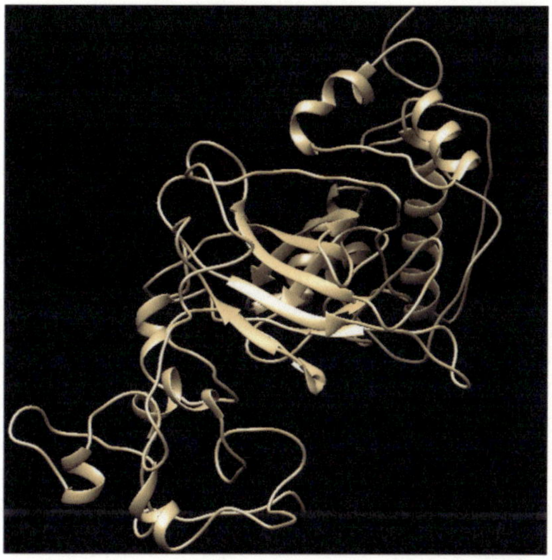

**Figure 1.**
*TP53 monomer (PDB ID 8F2I).*

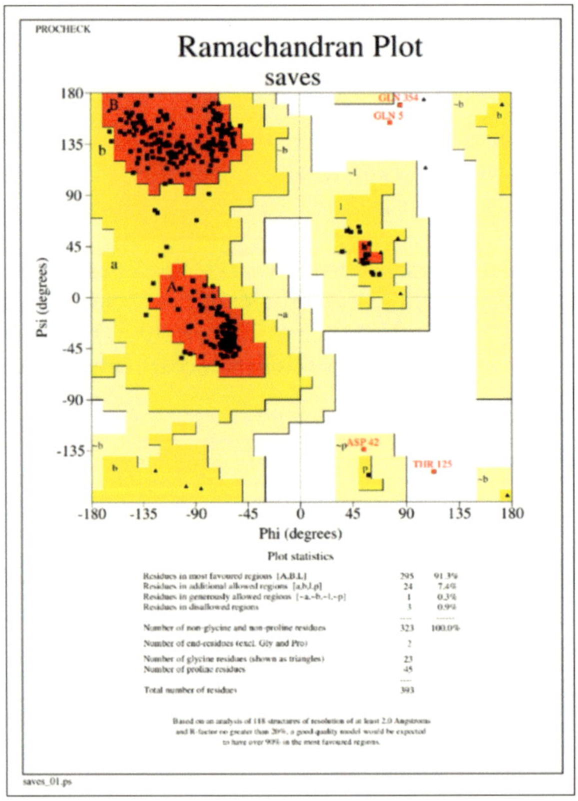


**Figure 2.**
*Ramachandran plot diagram.*

| Regions of the Ramachandran plot | Mutant tp53 |
|---|---|
| Allowed Regions: | |
| percentage of residues in most favored region | 92.3 |
| Percentage of residues in additionally allowed regions | 5.9 |
| Percentage of residues in generously allowed region | 1.2 |
| Percentage of residues in disallowed region | 0.6 |

**Table 2.**
*Residues of the generated mutant p53 models in the Ramachandran plot showing the quality of the modeled secondary structures.*

## 2.5 Binding sites and molecular docking

The built homology 3D models were utilized for molecular docking. In the first instance, the binding sites were found from the latest publication that recommended a new druggable pocket in the DNA-binding region of the mutant TP53. This pocket consists of the following amino acid residues: Arg174, glu 180, Glu192, his 193, Asp207, Asp208, Arg209, Asn210, Thr211, Phe212, Arg213, and His214 [20]. The tertiary structure of the protein was further predicted with the Prankweb server (https://prankweb.cz/) to predict the active binding sites present in the TP53 mutated protein as shown in **Figure 4**.

| Functions | Validation | Mutated TP53 model (%) |
|---|---|---|
| ERRAT | Overall Quality Factor | 85.24 |
| Verify3d | Status | Pass |
| | Residues has averaged 3D-1D score > = 0.1 | 87.79 |
| | amino acids have scored > = 0.1 in the 3D/1D profile | greater than 80% |
| Procheck | Ramachandran Plot | 92.3 |

**Table 3.**
*Results of the structure validation by different functions of SAVES.*

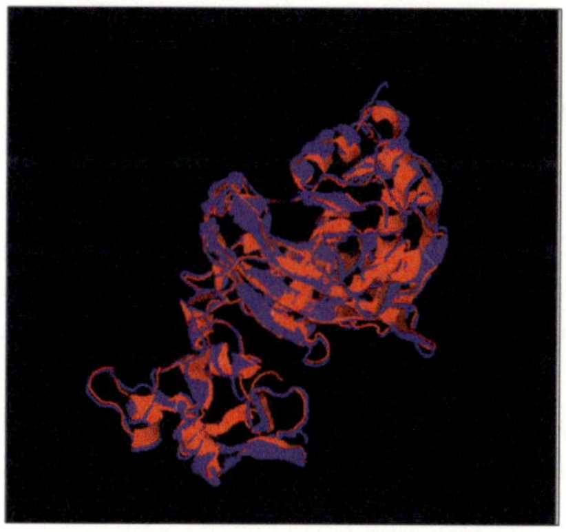

**Figure 3.**
*Visualization of superposition of two proteins (Protein-1(PDB 8FI) in blue and Protein-2 (T 53 mutated model in red).*

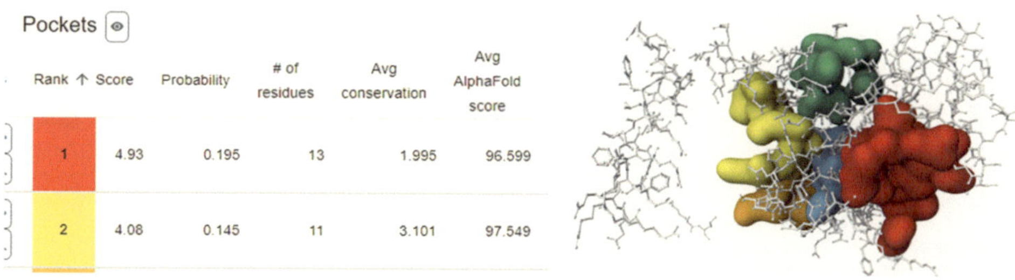


**Figure 4.**
*The two most probable binding sites with the highest probability is pocket 1 and 2 with a total of 24 residues.*

## 2.6 Molecular docking

A library of FDA-approved drugs (1123 compounds) (https://enamine.net/compound-libraries/bioactive-libraries/fda-approved-drugs-collection) was downloaded in SDF format and screened for initial virtual screening against the mutation c238y. Virtual screening is a computational technique used to search libraries of small molecules to distinguish those structures that have the highest probability to bind to a drug. Structure-based virtual screening (SBVS), also known as target-based virtual screening (TBVS), attempts to predict the best interaction between ligands against a molecular target to form a complex.

Prankweb binding-identified pockets were taken into consideration with the above residues' sites, which were used to confine the search space for virtual screening. Virtual screening was then performed on the mutated TP53 and 1123 FDA approved drugs using Dockey SoftwarE and PyRX 0.8. Dockey (https://github.com/lmdu/) is a novel tool to help in easing the accomplishment of molecular docking. Dockey combines several external tools (autodock vina) to implement the complete docking pipeline covering molecular sanitization, molecular preparation, interaction, and visualities. PyRx 0.8 (https://pyrx.sourceforge.io/) is a virtual screening tool for Computer-Aided Drug Discovery (CADD) that can be used to screen libraries of compounds against potential drug targets. The binding affinity for each FDA drug with the mutant TP53 with a more negative score of a compound signifies a higher binding capability.

The first 10 compounds with the largest binding affinities were chosen for additional analysis. The top 10 docking poses are depicted in **Tables 4** and **5**.

The Autodock Vina tool predicts the binding affinities of the first conformations, with zero RMSD values considered. No sets of controls were included in this study as no drugs were found to bind to this specific mutation. Given that there was no source point to make a comparison with the binding energy, drugs showing the lowest binding energies were taken for further investigation. For enhanced refinement in the *in silico* results, docking with Autodock 4.2.6 program (http: autodock.scripps.edu) was performed for the top four compounds. Umbralisib was withdrawn by the FDA from the market due to its toxicity. Hence, docking of the three compounds with mutated TP53 c238y was performed indigenously by docking one compound at a time to the mutated TP53 manually using Autodock 4.2.6 incorporated in AMDOCK. Autodock 4.2.6 was used to determine the lowest binding energies and ranked according to their binding affinities. AMDock (Assisted Molecular Docking) is an easy software for docking of protein-ligand complexes using AutoDock Vina and AutoDock 4.2.6.

| Ligand | Affinity | logKi | LE | Ki |
|---|---|---|---|---|
| Umbralisib_ | −10.09 | −7.396 | 0.24 | 40.17 nM |
| Ubrogepant | −9.336 | −6.843 | 0.233 | 143.42 nM |
| Maraviroc | −9.146 | −6.704 | 0.247 | 197.65 nM |
| Tolvaptan | −8.606 | −6.308 | 0.269 | 491.72 nM |
| Tucatinib | −8.678 | −6.361 | 0.241 | 435.45 nM |
| Zafirlukast | −8.33 | −6.106 | 0.203 | 783.48 nM |
| Zavegepant_ | −9.737 | −7.137 | 0.207 | 72.89 nM |
| Midostaurin | −9.916 | −7.269 | 0.231 | 53.89 nM |
| Paritaprevir_ | −8.668 | −6.354 | 0.188 | 442.87 nM |
| Atovastatin | −9.763 | −7.156 | 0.349 | 69.76 nM |

**Table 4.**
*Top 10 compounds obtained from virtual screening.*

| S/N | Receptor | Ligand | Affinity | lRMSD | uRMSD | logKi | LE | Ki |
|---|---|---|---|---|---|---|---|---|
| 1 | MutC238Y | Umbralisib | −10.28 | 0 | 0 | −7.535 | 0.245 | 29.15 nM |
| 2 | mutC238Y | Midostaurin | −9.947 | 0 | 0 | −7.291 | 0.231 | 51.14 nM |
| 3 | mutEC238Y | atovastatin | −9.393 | 0 | 0 | −6.885 | 0.335 | 130.27 nM |
| 4 | mutC238Y | Zavegepant | −9.594 | 0 | 0 | −7.032 | 0.204 | 92.79 nM |

**Table 5.**
*Top 4 compounds with the highest binding energy.*

## 3. Validation of molecular docking

The RMSD is a good method of Validation of Molecular Docking to split the ligand from its target and repeat docking in the same area, where the ligand was found previously. As such, we can easily analyze if the ligand and the same docked ligand are intersecting or not, through the value of parameter RMSD. Overall, 2 Å RMSD value for a conformation is considered a docking success.

### 3.1 Protein-ligand interaction profiler

PLIP (projects.biotec.tu-dresden.de/plip-web) is an internet-based server that gives analysis of protein-ligand interactions. PLIP detects hydrogen bonds, hydrophobic contacts between ligands and targets. The main target is to locate interactions in the dock complex. Hydrogen bonds and hydrophobic interactions play a vital role in revealing the specificity of drug candidates, with the active site residues of the target protein impacting the binding affinity and steadiness of the ligand–protein complex.

UCSF chimera (https://www.cgl.ucsf.edu/chimera) is a computer software for interactive visualization and analysis of molecular structures and sequence alignment. The option matchmaker is used as a validation method to calculate RMSD values of the three drugs: midostaurin, atorvastatin and zavegepant.

| Gene | Drug | Docking program | Docking software | Binding affinity (kcal/mol) | RMSD lb./up | RMSD(Å) |
|---|---|---|---|---|---|---|
| tp53mutated | midostaurin | Dockey virtual screening | vina | −9.94 | 0 | |
| | | Pyrx virtual Screening | vina | −9.92 | 0 | |
| | | Chimera 1.8 | | | | 1.82 Å |
| *Target* | *Drug* | *Docking Program* | *Docking Software* | *Binding affinity (kcal/mol)* | *KI* | *Ligand efficiency (LE)* |
| | | AMDOCK | Autock4.2.6 | −9.52 | 183.52 Nm | −0.23 |

**Table 6.**
*Docking analysis of midostaurin.*

### 3.2 Results and validation of molecular docking

Docking techniques are usually a way to find out large libraries of compounds such as drugs at a reasonable cost. The major limitations are the deficiency or limited protein flexibility. A combination of various docking procedures were used to screen drug database (**Tables 6–8**).

### 3.3 Interaction of the 3 ligands with mutated TP53

See **Table 9**.

| **Target** | **Drug** | **Docking program** | **Docking software** | **Binding affinity (kcal/mol)** | **RMSD lb./up** | **RMSD(Å)** |
|---|---|---|---|---|---|---|
| Mutated tp53 | atorvastatin | dockey VS | Vina | −9.39 | 0 | |
| | | Pyrx virtual Screening | Vina | −9.38 | 0 | |
| | | Chimera 1.8 | | | | 1.28 Å |
| *Target* | *Drug* | *Docking Program* | *Docking Software* | *Binding affinity (kcal/mol)* | *KI* | *Ligand efficiency (LE)* |
| | | AMDOCK | Autock4.2.6 | −7.19 | 5.37 μM | −0.22 |

**Table 7.**
*Docking analysis of atovastatin.*

| **Target** | **Drug** | **Docking program** | **Docking software** | **Binding affinity (kcal/mol)** | **RMSD lb./up** | **RMSD(Å)** |
|---|---|---|---|---|---|---|
| tp53mutated | Zavegepant | Dockey virtual screening | vina | 9.59 | 0 | |
| | | Pyrx virtual Screening | vina | −9.59 | 0 | |
| | | Chimera 1.8 | | | | 1.57 Å |
| *Target* | *Drug* | *Docking Program* | *Docking Software* | *Binding affinity (kcal/mol)* | *KI* | *Ligand efficiency (LE)* |
| | | AMDOCK | Autock4.2.6 | −9.93 | 52.63 Nm | −0.23 |

**Table 8.**
*Docking analysis of zavegepant.*

| Compound | Interacting amino acid residues | Number of hydrogen bonds |
|---|---|---|
| Midostaurin | 131A ASN, 373A LYS | 2 |
| Atovastatin | 271A GLU, 373A LYS, 131A ASN | 3 |
| Zavegepant | 111 A LEU, 351A LYS, 354A GLN, 359A PRO, 363A ARG, 371A SER, 373ALYS | 8 |

**Table 9.**
*Interactions of ligands.*

## 4. Discussion

As per this report above, the scenario of uterine leiomyosarcoma was described. This histology signifies a very rare tumor type where the ideal treatment is not available. Current antitumor protocols are not capable to cure patients with ULMS. Conventional anticancer drugs were used for treatment of the patient. Mutation of TP53, as occurs in ULMS, not only abrogates the P53 protein's normal tumor-suppressive function but also may disrupt cellular regulatory networks. At that time, personal genomic profiling was not performed, but the patient pursued the conventional route; hence, new treatment options are urgently needed. As at now, there are no effective therapeutic means to target (mutated) TP53. A novel concept in personalized oncology is tumor sequencing to discover patient-specific mutations that can be tackled by targeted drugs. NGS sequencing information can be used to identify new therapies for individual patients by using virtual screening method. The mutation in a leiomyosarcoma patient has been used as an example that proved the viability of this concept. The investigation was concentrated on examining FDA-approved drugs, since repurposing of drugs initially approved for diseases other than cancer provided interesting treatment options for many patients. The mutation obtained by genomic profiling of the patient's tumor has several consequences for treatment.

The sequencing of genomic profiling provides information on driver mutation. Proper interpretation of the mutational analysis is desirable to make concise decisions, to understand which mutations are most appropriate for virtual drug screening. As a result, it can be considered to search for drugs that have already been approved for other diseases showing anti-cancer activity. This concept is commonly known as drug repurposing and has proven to be a success.

NGS sequencing data were obtained from blood CTDNA to identify mutations. The mutations are screened against already FDA-approved drugs that bound with high affinity to mutated proteins in a ULMS patient. A database of 1123 FDA-approved drugs was first screened by PyRX software and Dockey software. The results obtained were further refined by molecular docking with AutoDock 4.2.6. Virtual drug screening unraveled a panel of drugs that bound with high affinity to TP53-mutated c238y, which is the main driver mutation. These drugs were from various classes and had different pharmaco-dynamic and pharmaco-kinetic activities. The drugs identified by this virtual screening uncovered anti-lipid (atovastatin) umbrasilib used for rare forms of refractory lymphoma; midostaurin for high-risk acute myeloid leukemia (AML), and zavegepant for acute treatment of migraine. The issue was which drug would be more beneficial for this ULMS patient.

Umbralisib, a kinase inhibitor for PI3K-delta and casein kinase CK1-epsilon, has been approved for the treatment of relapsing and refractory marginal cell lymphoma and follicular lymphoma. Umbralisib was withdrawn from the market due to safety concerns as the drug was associated with a possible increased risk of death. Therefore, umbrasilib will not be considered for drug repurposing in this specific case.

Midostaurin (as Rydapt) is a multitarget kinase inhibitor that was initially characterized as a potential broad-spectrum antineoplastic agent, with activity toward diverse solid and hematopoietic tumors. It has shown to increase the overall survival rate in patients with AML as an adjunct therapy along with chemotherapeutic agents. It targets multiple WT and mutated kinases that, when activated, constitutively stimulate aberrant signaling cascades that lead to malignancies such as AML. Midostaurin is therapeutically beneficial as a combination therapy for patients undergoing chemotherapy. It potently inhibits multiple receptor tyrosine kinases VEGFR2, KIT, and PDGFR and WT tyrosine kinases. The patient also had a PDGFRA mutation, which can be targeted by midostaurin. PDGFRA is involved in tumor angiogenesis and maintenance of the tumor microenvironment and is implicated in metastasis, as well as playing a role in normal angiogenesis. Hence, midostaurin can be combined with other drugs to target both mutated TP53 and PDGFRA.

Zavegepant is a calcitonin gene-related peptide (CGRP) receptor antagonist. CGRP is released from sensory nerves and acts as a strong vasodilator. Zavegepant is a third-generation CGRP receptor antagonist that is small and highly soluble. Due to its pharmacological properties, it can be administered intranasally. In March 2023, the FDA approved the use of zavegepant nasal spray for the acute treatment of migraine. This is a useful adjunct for this patient to take this drug intranasally to target the lung metastasis.

Atorvastatin (Lipitor®) is a lipid-lowering drug included in the statin class of medication statins and is considered standard practice for patients following any cardiovascular event. Preclinical data from University of Kansas Cancer Center showed that several statins, like atorvastatin, suppressed mutated Tp53 level and cell growth selectively (PMID: 27775703). The trial tested whether atorvastatin can selectively suppress the level of conformationally mutant p53 protein in subjects with resectable tumors or previously treated acute myeloid leukemia (AML) at dose of 80 mg/day orally for 1–4 weeks using a 141 gene NGS panel, including TP53 (Clinical trial identification: NCT03560882). At this juncture, this shows that computational methods with *in silico* analysis can predict drugs for rare tumor treatment. When these results were obtained, the leiomyosarcoma patient was already at a deteriorative state despite aggressive treatments. Unfortunately, the patient died on 9 July 2024 before any recommendation of an individualized treatment with the above repurposed drugs could be implemented. Hence, a final proof of the clinical success of this computational method presented in this study could not be given. Nevertheless, the study represents a preclinical viable approach to identify possible treatment candidates in cases that lack therapeutic options, which is a scenario frequently occurring in clinical oncology. Repurposing of approved FDA drugs may not deliver more drugs for the individual treatment of cancer patients due to the multiplicity of tumor-related mutations. The identified drugs may be used as a starting point for further drug development to improve ULMS therapy in the future. The three drugs above can be combined safely to increase survival and to block progression of the disease. Despite the attractiveness of the virtual drug screening approach based on tumor sequencing data, there are also some limitations of this approach that have to be addressed. Virtual drug screening of FDA-approved drug may result in the identification of a certain rate of false positive candidates. Therefore, results from virtual drug screening should be validated by *in vitro* or *in vivo* experiments and in clinical settings.

## 5. Conclusion

Genomic repurposing may expose drug candidates for the advance improvement of personalized treatment in cancer. A combination of tumor genomic profiling and virtual screening method can identify new repurpose drug. FDA-approved drugs can aid in making appropriate compound predictions to inhibit mutated proteins and to enhance cancer therapy for each patient. ULMS tumor entity is unresponsive to standard chemotherapy and radiotherapy (which may exacerbate metastasis), and effective treatment of the disease are scarce. At this juncture, a way to discover other protocol of this rare tumor is warranted. For this reason, genomic sequencing of the ULMS tumor was performed using NGS analysis. Using computational software, three FDA-approved drugs, which are not routinely used for ULMS treatment, were identified. These compounds could be useful in circumstances that the conventional treatment have failed. The repurposing concept can be used for ULMS as well as for other rare refractory resistant tumors. This concept is coined as targeted computational-guided drug repurposing method, signifying an original prospect for personalized tumor therapy that warrants further research.

## Contribution

I would like to thank Ms. Mansourah Hosany for proofreading countless pages and correcting the manuscript of this paper.

## Funding

No funding was provided for this publication.

## Conflict of interest

The author declares there is no conflict of interest.

## Compliance with ethical standards

Informed written consent had been given by the patient that the data are allowed to be scientifically used and published (dated: April 26, 2024).

## Author details

Hoosdally Shakeel
Department of Chemistry, Ministry of Tertiary Education and Scientific Research, Mauritius

*Address all correspondence to: shoosdally@moemu.org

## References

[1] Siegel RL, Miller KD, Fuchs HE, Jemal A. Cancer statistics, 2022. CA: A Cancer Journal for Clinicians. 2022;**72**:7-33. DOI: 10.3322/caac.21708

[2] von Konow A, Ghanei I, Styring E, Hainaut L. Late local recurrence and metastasis in soft tissue sarcoma of the extremities and trunk wall: Better outcome after treatment of late events compared with early. Annals of Surgical Oncology. 2021;**28**:7891-7902. DOI: 10.1245/s10434-021-09942-8

[3] Ognjanovic S, Olivier M, Bergemann TL, Hainaut P. Sarcomas in TP53 germline mutation carriers: A review of the IARC TP53 database. Cancer. 2012;**118**:1387-1396. DOI: 10.1002/cncr.26390

[4] Blaye C, Kind M, Stoeckle E, Brouste V, Kantor G, Le Loarer F, et al. Local and metastatic relapse features in patients after a primary soft tissue sarcoma: Advocating for a better-tailored follow-up. Frontiers in Oncology. 2019;**9**:559. DOI: 10.3389/fonc.2019.00559

[5] Penel N et al. Testing new regimens in patients with advanced soft tissue sarcoma: Analysis of publications from the last 10 years. Annals of Oncology. 2011;**22**:1266-1272

[6] Cantero MM, Sepúlveda JM, D'Haene N, Gutiérrez-Guamán MJ, Rodríguez Á, de Lope C, et al. TP53, ATRX alterations, and low tumor mutation load feature IDH-wildtype giant cell glioblastoma despite exceptional ultra-mutated tumors. Neuro-Oncology Advances. 2020;**2**(1):vdz0

[7] Claussin C, Chang M. The many facets of homologous recombination at telomeres. Microbial Cell. 2015;**2**(9):308-321. DOI: 10.15698/mic2015.09.224. Available from: https://pmc.ncbi.nlm.nih.gov/articles/PMC5354574/

[8] Farshid G, Pradhan M, Goldblum J, Weiss SW. Leiomyosarcoma of somatic soft tissues: A tumor of vascular origin with multivariate analysis of outcome in 42 cases. The American Journal of Surgical Pathology. 2002;**26**:14-24

[9] Mbatani N, Olawaiye AB, Prat J. Uterine sarcomas. International Journal of Gynaecology and Obstetrics. 2018;**143**(Suppl. 2):51-58

[10] Gladdy RA, Qin L-X, Moraco N, Agaram NP, Brennan MF, Singer S. Predictors of survival and recurrence in primary leiomyosarcoma. Annals of Surgical Oncology. 2013;**20**:1851-1857

[11] Gustafson P, Willén H, Baldetorp B, Fernö M, Akerman M, Rydholm A. Soft tissue leiomyosarcoma. A population-based epidemiologic and prognostic study of 48 patients, including cellular DNA content. Cancer. 1992;**70**:114-119

[12] Toro JR, Travis LB, Wu HJ, Zhu K, Fletcher CDM, Devesa SS. Incidence patterns of soft tissue sarcomas, regardless of primary site, in the surveillance, epidemiology and end results program, 1978-2001: An analysis of 26,758 cases. International Journal of Cancer. 2006;**119**:2922-2930

[13] Toro JR, Travis LB, Wu HJ, Zhu K, Fletcher CDM, Devesa SS. Incidence patterns of soft tissue sarcomas, regardless of primary site, in the surveillance, epidemiology and end results program, 1978-2001: An analysis of 26,758. International Journal of Cancer. 15 Dec 2006;**15**(2):2922-2930. Available

from: https://pubmed.ncbi.nlm.nih.gov/17013893/

[14] Verweij J, Lee SM, Ruka W, Buesa J, Coleman R, van Hoessel R, et al. Randomized phase II study of docetaxel versus doxorubicin in first- and second-line chemotherapy for locally advanced or metastatic soft tissue sarcomas in adults: A study of the European Organization for Research and Treatment of cancer soft tissue and bone sarcoma group. Journal of Clinical Oncology. 2000;**18**:2081-2086

[15] Lazzari G, Buono G, Zannino B, Silvano G. Breast cancer adjuvant radiotherapy in BRCA1/2, TP53, ATM genes mutations: Are there solved issues? Breast Cancer. **13**:299-310. Available from: https://pubmed.ncbi.nlm.nih.gov/34012291/

[16] Kadioglu O, Efferth T. Contributions from emerging transcriptomics technologies and computational strategies for drug discovery. Investigational New Drugs. 2014;**32**(6):1316-1319

[17] Sirota M et al. Discovery and preclinical validation of drug indications using compendia of public gene expression data. Science Translational Medicine. 2011;**3**(96):96ra77\

[18] Imako GK, Wintrob ZA, Sulik DA, Donato JL, Ceacareanu AC. Synergistic benefit of statin and metformin in gastrointestinal malignancies. Journal of Pharmacy Practice. 2017;**2**:185-194. pii: 0897190015627255. Available from: https://pubmed.ncbi.nlm.nih.gov/26811340/

[19] Levine AJ, Lane DP, editors. The p53 Family. Cold Spring Harbor Perspectives in Biology. Cold Spring Harbor, N.Y: Cold Spring Harbor Laboratory Press; 2010. ISBN 978-0-87969-830-027. Availabe from: https://www.cshlpress.com/default.tpl?cart=17323024452241027250&fromlink=T&linkaction=full&linksortby=oop_title&--eqSKUdatarq=864

[20] Pradhan MR, Siau JW, Kannan S, Nguyen MN. Simulations of mutant p53 DNA binding domains reveal a novel druggable pocket. Nucleic Acids Research. 2019;**47**(4):1637-1652. DOI: 10.1093/nar/gky1314

Chapter 2

# Ovarian Cancer Screening

*Abubakr Mohamed Ali Nasr*


## Abstract

Ovarian cancer screening remains elusive in spite of the tireless efforts. The challenges faced include the prevalence of ovarian cancer and its impact on the positive predictive value of screening tests. Effective screening is highly needed in view of being the deadliest gynecological cancer with late presentation. The diversity of targeted population, low and high risk as well as the ambiguity in oncogenesis and shared origin by fallopian tubes and peritoneum are genuine obstacles in unifying a screening program for the heterogenous disease. The consensus does not recommend screening in low-risk populations. Evaluation of available screening tests in multiple trials did not prove reduction in mortality. There may be an increase in detection of early disease. However, the impact on mortality and quality of life is questionable. The screening tests including pelvic sonography, tumor markers, proteoms, mRNA, free DNA and symptom-based screening did not prove significant statistical power in view of the risky diagnostic testing with laparoscopy and significant possibility of false positive results. There is potential role for developments in the available tests and future developments including AI.


**Keywords:** ovarian cancer, screening, pelvic sonography, CA125, proteoms, mRNA, symptom-based screening, ovary, oncogenesis, tumour makers, BRCA mutation

## 1. Introduction

Ovarian cancer screening programs have been an unbeatable challenge despite great efforts using multiple pathways to achieve a successful, cost-effective, reproducible outcome model that can be implemented in clinical practice.

The classical screening model of ovarian cancer screening applied to current clinical practice basically includes CA125 and transvaginal ultrasound (TVS) as screening tools. Clinical symptoms, biomarkers, and genetic testing have been suggested as screening tools as well.

The targeted screening population characteristics have been an area of debate as the effectiveness of the tools is affected by the low incidence of the disease. So, targeting an asymptomatic population or those with risk factors or genetic predisposition is unlikely to be tested with the same tools from a cost-efficacy point of view.

The processes of screening, early detection, and assessment of malignancy risk in an incidental ovarian/adnexal mass are intersected domains. It is crucial that



IntechOpen

boundaries need to be clarified when addressing such scenarios in clinical practice. The intersections are due to the similar tools used in assessment, which are TVS, CA 125, and biomarkers.

The current recommendation by most reputable bodies in gynecology does not recommend screening for ovarian cancer in a normal population. There is some dispute on high-risk groups. This recommendation is based on the finding that screening did not prove to reduce mortality; moreover, the screened population is subjected to significant hazards from interventions based on screening results.

## 2. Basic screening concepts

The concept of health overrides the clinical practice of disease treatment, aiming for a better quality of care and life. The screening programs fitted widely in health and medical practice. In gynecology, a successful model is cervical screening programs.

Screening simply means seeing the unseen. The tools for detection need to be sensitive and specific for the best efficacy of the intended screening program. This is demonstrated by the iceberg phenomenon of disease.

The screening program as a whole is composed of screening tests and preventive actions. It is crucial to discriminate between screening programs and screening tests. Screening programs may include disease prevention measures as well. Screening tests are intended to pick a high-risk group for the screened condition who will be subsequently subjected to a diagnostic test. An example of this scenario is CA125 as a screening test and histopathology as a diagnostic test. The triad of screening programs is screening tests, the disease tested for, and the preventive measure taken or offered. The screening discriminatory power refers to the ability of the test to accurately categorize groups of the tested population. The detection rate of a screening test refers to the number of populations who tested positive according to the screening test, irrespective of being affected or not. The screening discriminatory power is related to the detection rate. The screening and diagnostic tests are statistically correlated. Important terms to be clearly understood are true positive, true negative, false positive, and false negative. These categories will generate important statistical values in screening, which are positive predictive and negative predictive values of screening tests. Positive predictive value is the possibility of being affected "true positive" when tested positive according to the screening test [1].

The basic concepts in statistical definitions of validity of screening/diagnostic tests are mandatory for interpretation of screening tools to be discussed.

**Table 1** explains the basic definition of screening/diagnostic test principles. These include

| | **Truth (gold standard)** | |
|---|---|---|
| **Result** | **Disease present** | **Disease absent** |
| Positive | True Positive a | False Positive b |
| Negative | False Positive c | True Negative d |

**Table 1.**
*Statistic values of screening tests.*

- Sensitivity
- Specificity
- Positive predictive value
- Negative predictive value
- Prevalence = True Positives (a + c)

Total Population (a + b + c + d)

- Sensitivity is the ability of a test to correctly classify an individual as diseased = True Positive/True Positive + False Negative *100
    - (a/a + c) *100
- Specificity is the ability of a test to correctly classify an individual as disease-free = True Negative/True negative + False Positive *100
    - (d/b + d) *100
- Positive predictive value (PPV) refers to the ability of the screening test to pick the truly affected.
- Negative predictive value (NPV) refers to the ability of the screening test to exclude those who are not affected.
- The prevalence of the condition tested in a population affects PPV and NPV. The PPV is positively related to prevalence, while the NPV is inversely related to the prevalence of the condition tested.
- The Gold Standard Test is the definitive diagnostic test, such as histopathology in ovarian cancer.

Performance of a screening program is measured in terms of discriminatory power and predictive value. Those with positive screening results will have their risk increased by the ratio of determined risk (sensitivity) over the false-positive rate (specificity), a factor known as the likelihood ratio. Discriminatory power is not easy to compute for progressive diseases such as gynecologic cancer. The preclinical state and length of follow-up affect the detection rate [1].

The screening in a progressive disease is not synonymous with acute disease. In the case of progressive disease, there are two possibilities. The ability to advance the diagnosis is the best option. If not achievable, the second option is early detection of the early stages of the disease. The central question is whether early diagnosis will improve prognosis. The relationship between screening program efficacy and long survival due to early diagnosis is subjected to two powerful biases. The first is lead time bias, and the second is length bias. Financial costs and benefits of screening programs are evaluated by calculating the unit cost of each component of the screening process. This depends on the statistical values discussed in the previous section.

Sensitivity analysis can be adjusted to determine what aspects of the screening program are most price-sensitive. In medical practice, provision of care for diseased is different from provision of screening for healthy and possibly diseased. Since screening is a proactive intervention, those who are not true positives are subjected to further unnecessary testing and interventions with possible significant hazards and financial and psychological burdens. The health care providers of screening tests are expected to provide adequate counseling to ensure that the one receiving screening tests is fully informed and able to make sound choices. This needs counseling tools more than the face-to-face traditional approach, such as infographics and video materials [1].

Criteria for implementing a screening program for a specific disease include:

- The disease significantly impacts health.
- The disease has an intermediate to high probability of occurrence in a population.
- A critical point for disease detection must exist.
- Medical care is available if the screening is positive.
- Patients are willing and able to undergo further evaluation and treatment.

The United States Preventive Services Task Force (USPSTF) recommends against screening for ovarian cancer in asymptomatic women. This is based on the finding that ovarian cancer screening in asymptomatic women did not reduce the risk of ovarian cancer-related death in the screened population. The second point considered in stating this recommendation is the excess risks and complications associated with the false screening results. Those who tested positive will be subjected to surgical intervention in the form of laparoscopy or laparotomy. These surgical procedures are intended to confirm the diagnosis and treat the disease. The hazards associated with the current screening for ovarian cancer using the currently adopted tools are considered moderate [2]. The analogy of screening programs in asymptomatic women cannot be replicated in women with ovarian masses, genetic predisposition, or family history of ovarian cancer. This needs to be addressed when discussing screening tests in subsequent sections.

## 3. Magnitude of ovarian cancer

The lifetime risk of ovarian cancer is around 1.4%, which equals 1 in 71 according to US statistics. Ovarian cancer is a deadly disease with a lifetime risk of death due to invasive ovarian malignancy, approximately 1 in 95. Although ovarian cancer is not common among women (3% among American women), its rank is the top gynecologic cancer and the 5th top of all cancers leading to death in women. Most ovarian cancer is reported in women above 55 years. Only one-third is below 55 years. Most ovarian cancers are diagnosed with advanced disease (stage III or IV). Women with advanced disease constitute two-thirds when diagnosed. Moreover, most women present late with nonspecific symptoms. The delay in diagnosis and advance diagnosis add to the poor outcome. There is evidence that early diagnosis of ovarian cancer is associated with a 90% 5-year survival rate. In case of advanced disease, the 5-year survival rate drops to 33%. The extent of major surgery and its associated morbidity in advanced disease compared to conservative surgery in early invite genuine efforts for early detection. It is prudent to consider quality of life and fertility issues when ovarian cancer is detected early, especially in young women [3].

### 3.1 Ovarian carcinogenesis

As mentioned in the previous section, components of screening include disease testing and preventive action. Implementation of screening tests should address the disease process in all aspects that affect the screening program.

Ovarian cancer is the most lethal gynecologic malignancy worldwide. The median age of diagnosis is 63 years. The lifetime risk of ovarian cancer in the general population is 1–2%. Approximately 90% of ovarian cancer develops from surface epithelial cells.

Historically, it was thought that high-grade ovarian cancer developed from the ovarian surface epithelium due to error in cell replication associated with repair and trauma caused by ovulation [4, 5].

There is compelling evidence that most high-grade serous carcinomas arise from the distal fallopian tube and not from the ovary, from serous tubal intraepithelial carcinoma [6].

Although ovarian cancer fits the criteria for screening, being a fatal disease, available and possibly effective treatment in an early stage, features of ovary and ovarian cancer development complicate the screening process, rendering its efficacy. The transition between early stages and late stages is unclear. There is no precursor lesion to detect. The presence of a precursor lesion at an accessible location will allow detection of early invasive disease. The best example is cervical cancer screening. The disease may be of diffuse origin as well, from multiple sites in the peritoneal cavity. The embryological development of the ovary and the different cell lines, as well as the relationship of the peritoneum to the epithelial covering of the ovary, need to be addressed in the conceptual frame to understand the complicated oncogenesis process in epithelial ovarian cancer. Most of the ovarian cancers occur in women above the age of 50 as sporadic cases, with 10% of cases being related to genetic and familial risk factors. These issues need to be considered upon implementing screening tests in order to achieve the statistical values that will enable a cost-effective, safe program with a "positive predictive value of 10%" [3].

The correlation of the results of recent molecular genetic studies with clinical and histopathologic findings pointed toward a new model for ovarian carcinogenesis. The model for ovarian carcinogenesis proposed by R.J. Kurman suggests that ovarian carcinogenesis can be divided into two groups. The model suggested categorizes borderline tumors as type one. Type two refers to the rapidly growing aggressive type of ovarian cancer. Borderline ovarian tumors are considered tumors of low malignant potential. The histological subtypes include micropapillary serous, mucinous, endometrioid, and clear cell carcinomas. From a genetic point of view, this group is genetically stable compared to the type II group. There may be mutations in a number of genes. Type II is characterized by genetic mutations in *TP53*. The histological subtype of the type II model includes high-grade serous and mucinous carcinomas, carcinosarcomas, and undifferentiated carcinomas. Being so different hinders the application of the same screening tool for both models. Precursor lesions may be identified in type I, which is not the case in the type II model [7].

According to the above-mentioned features, the detection rate for screening tests applied in type I is likely to be more successful compared to the type II model. Since screening and early detection may not be feasible for the type II model, the next checkpoint is the detection of low-volume disease. However, the prognostic value of low volume detection on survival and quality of life is an area of dispute. In addition to the two models' form suggested and its impact on screening potentials, the origin, spread, and transit time between early and late stages are factors to be considered. These factors, in addition to anatomical differences, make the analogy between ovarian and cervical cancers illogical. The transit time from precursor lesions to invasive disease in ovarian cancer may be short compared to the scenario in cervical cancer. The spread of high-grade ovarian cancer "type II model" may occur early in the disease process. There is evidence supporting extra-ovarian origin in ovarian cancer as well as multiple origins. The possible sites of extra-ovarian origin include the fallopian tube and primary peritoneal cancers. Addressing prophylactic oophorectomy in women with BRCA 1 and BRCA 2 mutations enables better understanding the possibility of extra-ovarian origin of "ovarian" cancers. In reality, some ovarian cancer cases are primary peritoneal or fallopian tube cancers. The study on prophylactic salpingo-oophorectomy and the risk of ovarian, fallopian tube, and peritoneal cancer in women with BRCA1 and BRCA2 mutations detected 32 cases of ovarian cancer in intact ovaries. At the time of prophylactic surgery, 11 cancers were detected. After prophylactic oophorectomy, seven cases were diagnosed. Over 20 years following prophylactic oophorectomy, the cumulative risk of developing peritoneal cancer is 4.3%. The risk reduction of ovarian cancer achieved with bilateral oophorectomy is 80%. This demonstrated that oophorectomy will not eliminate the risk of developing "ovarian" cancer [7, 8].

The relationship between the fallopian tube fimbria and ovarian cancer has been addressed extensively. Paul van Diest studied the fallopian tubes of women with genetic predisposition to ovarian cancer, "BRCA1 and BRCA2." An interesting finding is the presence of dysplastic changes in the fallopian tubes studied. The histological dysplastic changes were related to modifications in cell cycle, apoptosis, and related proteins. This finding may invite innovative ideas to screen the fallopian tubes for such dysplastic changes or the corresponding molecular and cellular changes. The obstacle will be the anatomical site; however, development in hysteroscopy may allow future access to the endosalpinx and fallopian tube fimbria [9].

DW Kindelberger studied the proposed origins of pelvic serous carcinoma, which include the ovary, fallopian tube, and peritoneum. Fimbria has been identified as the site of origin for early serous carcinoma. Cases positive for endosalpinx, including fimbria, were classified as tubal, ovarian, or primary peritoneal in origin. Mutation in *p53* tested as well. Tubal intraepithelial carcinoma coexists in all forms of pelvic serous carcinoma and is a plausible origin for many of these tumors [10].

The heterogeneity of ovarian cancer in behavior and origin claims different approaches to detection and treatment. Innovations in screening tests for ovarian cancer and implementation of an effective ovarian cancer screening program mandate a solid, scientific, and sound understanding of ovarian carcinogenesis. The conceptual frame needs to address ovarian anatomy, genetics, and physiological processes.

## 4. Ovarian cancer screening obstacles

The current practice of serum assays of CA 125 and TVS as potential screening tests for ovarian cancer is not recommended in the general population. Even in a high-risk population, it has limited value. The screening test challenges include:

- The failure to identify a histologic precursor lesion.
- The failure to identify a molecular event that precedes malignant transformation.
- Low prevalence in the general population.
- The surgical morbidity associated with a positive screening test. For a clinically acceptable test, a positive predictive value of 10% is required; this means that for one case detected, 10 will undergo surgical procedure to confirm the diagnosis.
- The small number of true early-stage high carcinomas detected.

The goal of ovarian cancer screening is to detect disease when confined to the ovary. If ovarian cancer at its earliest recognizable stage is not confined to the ovary, this goal will be elusive [7].

Ovarian cancer screening associated risks include:

- Surgical interventions
- Overdiagnosis
- Psychological stress
- Financial burden

### 4.1 Screening tools/tests

In clinical practice, there should be clear demarcation between diagnostic and screening tests, as well as screening tests/tools and screening programs. In the case of multiple tests, the gold standard test for confirmation of diagnosis is considered a reference to give value for other tests. The gold standard test in ovarian cancer is the histology report. The diagnostic and screening tests include TVS, tumor markers and biomarkers, and index symptoms.

The improvement in detection rate of a specific test could be feasible due to multiple factors such as technical improvements, artificial intelligence, learning curve, and modification of algorithms adopted in test interpretation based on specific criteria.

### 4.2 Tumor marker: Cancer antigen 125

CA125 stands for "Carbohydrate 125" or more recently to "cancer antigen 125" is a mucinous glycoprotein on the surface of ovarian cancer cells. CA125 has been the most popular tumor marker used for management of ovarian cancer for the last four decades. The clinical uses of CA125 were mainly for risk assessment of malignancy index and treatment follow-up. The role as a screening test did not prove statistical significance to adopt as a screening test on its own. CA125 was first described by Best et al. in 1981, when a murine monoclonal antibody (OC125) was developed to react with each of six epithelial ovarian carcinoma cell lines [11]. CA125 expression is not peculiar to ovarian cancer. CA125 expression has been associated with benign and malignant conditions as well as non-oncologic conditions. The expression of

CA 125 has been documented in tissues derived from both coelomic and Mullerian epithelium. It is also expressed by epithelia of multiple internal organs, such as the stomach, pancreas, and lungs. Non-ovarian malignancies and benign and physiologic conditions such as pregnancy, menstruation, fibroids, and endometriosis were associated with elevated CA125. From a prognostic point of view, no correlation was found between expression of CA125 and tumor grade [12]. These findings reduce the value of elevated CA125 in screening ovarian cancer due to the high false-positive rate. The interventions built on a screening test with a high false-positive rate will impose unjustified risks on the screened population. Following positive screening, the algorithm will be directed toward diagnostic testing, which involves surgical interventions. The screening positive predictive value of CA125 is less than 10%. Such a positive predictive value is not accepted in clinical practice. In order to achieve a positive predictive value of 10%, a screening test for ovarian cancer (even with a 100% sensitivity) would require a minimum specificity of 99.6%. The statistical characteristics of CA125 as a screening test will not satisfy such criteria. CA125 is increased in less than 50% of early-stage ovarian cancer, while 20% of epithelial ovarian cancer may not express CA125. There may be a discrepancy between tissue and blood levels of CA125. In clinical practice, the measured CA125 is blood level. A false-negative result of serum CA125 has been clinically documented. This will reduce the screening potential more as true positive cases may be missed. Normal serum CA125 in cases of ovarian cancer may be due to a lack of expression of the antigen by tumor cells as well. The specificity of tissue CA125 to ovarian cancer is very high, as it may be detected in many tissues and conditions, unlike blood level, which is more specific to ovarian cancer with the mentioned limitations. It is crucial to differentiate between interpretation of CA125 blood level as a screening test, predictive test for women with masses, and prognostic test for follow-up of treatment in women with ovarian cancer. The menopausal state is another criterion to be considered upon interpretation of the CA125 test result. The statistical values are different in each category according to the study population.

SE Kabawat studied CA125 antigenic distribution, including fetal tissue. An interesting finding was that normal surface epithelial cells of fetal and adult ovaries fail to express CA125, despite the presence of antigen in normal mesothelial cells and in tumors that are thought to be derived from the ovarian surface epithelium. This finding suggests that, during normal development, ovarian surface epithelium acquires properties that are distinct from those of both mesothelium and Mullerian epithelium [13].

Other biomarkers have been recommended to improve sensitivity, specificity, and predictive values. CA125 remained the single best biomarker for epithelial ovarian cancer, as demonstrated by testing a panel of biomarkers that included CA125, HEA4, transthyretin, CA15.3, and CA72.4 in a randomized trial phase II and III of PLCO [14].

In an attempt to improve the detection rate of CA125, combinations of other markers such as HE4 (Human Epididymis 4) have been addressed. There is some evidence that the dual marker combination of CA125 and HE4 will improve sensitivity and specificity in predicting malignancy in women with pelvic masses. This may allow successful classification of patients into high- and low-risk groups [15]. Upon interpretation of the CA125 test result, the menopause state needs to be considered as the cutoff value affects the specificity and sensitivity of the test.

Ca125 blood level is measured as part of a prediction model for assessing malignancy risk in women with pelvic mass. The statistical values for detection rates will differ according to the level of CA125 used in the suggested risk index.

CA125 achieves a sensitivity of 78.3% and a specificity of 82% at a level of 35 U/mL. Increasing the cutoff level to 65 U/mL, the sensitivity decreased to 71.7% and the specificity increased to 92.5%. The Risk of Malignancy Index (RMI) is the most utilized algorithm for predicting malignancy in women with pelvic mass. The RMI utilizes CA125, menopause status, and pelvic sonography as parameters for obtaining a value. The calculated value will help decision-making for the clinical pathway. The options will be a gynecology oncology center, a gynecology oncology unit, or a general gynecology unit [16]. At a cutoff value of 200 for detection of epithelial ovarian cancer, the RMI algorithm reported a sensitivity of 87.4%, a specificity of 56.8%, a positive predictive value of 86.8%, and a negative predictive value of 58.1% [17].

To improve the sensitivity, specificity, and predictive values of CA124 in detecting ovarian cancer, risk calculation with serial CA125 measurements was compared to fixed CA125 measurements. Using serial measurements of CA125 improved the detection rate from 84 to 93%. This is a statistically significant improvement at the expense of the higher cost of serial CA125 testing. Adopting serial annual measurement of CA125 aiming for a PPV of 2% and specificity of 98%, preclinical detection sensitivity increases from 62 to 86%. To improve PPV, other tools, such as multiple levels of pelvic ultrasound, are required. As mentioned above, PPV of less than 10% is not clinically acceptable due to the unjustified hazards of screening-based interventions. So, preclinical detection of ovarian cancer using serial CA125 levels interpreted with the risk calculation significantly improves screening performance compared with a fixed cutoff for CA125 [18].

The interpretation of serum CA125 as a screening tool in a low-risk population is different from reading the value within a scenario of suspected ovarian malignancy. The value of CA125 interpretation in case of suspected malignancy is triaging the care provision under oncology center, unit, or general gynecology unit. CA125 can be elevated in conditions other than epithelial ovarian cancer. On the other hand, CA125 serum level is not increased in 50% of early-stage epithelial ovarian cancer. Beyond the scope of this chapter, CA125 plays an important role in monitoring patients with epithelial ovarian cancer who underwent different modalities of treatment. Although the same test is applied, the interpretation is different as the tested population is different.

### 4.3 Pelvis sonography

The first efforts to identify ovarian tumors using ultrasound were reported by Campbell et al. Interpretation of ovarian ultrasound mandates understanding basic anatomy of the ovary. The normal ovary is an ovoid structure. The normal ovary measures 3 cm x 2 cm x 2 cm, with an average volume of 10 $cm^3$. The ovary normally decreases in size after menopause as part of the changes taking place in the female reproductive organs. In premenopausal women, an ovarian volume less than 20 $cm^3$ is considered normal. The ovary is composed of an outer cortex and an inner medulla. The echogenicity of each layer is different. The position of the ovary is highly variable as it is connected to the uterus *via* the utero-ovarian ligament and the lateral pelvic wall *via* the infundibulopelvic ligament that carries the ovarian vessels and nerves [19].

Pelvic sonography, being safe and easy to use and interpret, represented a potentially promising screening tool for ovarian cancer. The screening potential increased with the development of technology and the resolution of machines used. The pelvic sonography can accurately give objective data about the structure and dimensions of the ovary and ovarian masses. Data about blood flow can be measured using Doppler mode.

Transvaginal ultrasound (TVS) evaluation of the ovary in the context of ovarian cancer screening has been addressed in four major trials. These include the Kentucky, PLCO, UKCTCOCS, and SCSOCS trials. The Kentucky, UKCTCOCS, and SCSOCS trials report a shift to early-stage detection. The Kentucky trial reports a survival benefit. An inherent feature of pelvic sonography is the lack of ability to diagnose ovarian cancer. It will merely describe the lesion detected. So, the benefits include detection and risk scoring. Further interventions are needed to confirm the diagnosis. The difficulty in risk scoring is more in early disease compared to late disease. A positive predictive value of 1.5% was obtained upon testing pelvic sonography as a screening test in 14,594 cases. Out of 67 cases tested positive, one proved to be primary ovarian cancer [20].

Current practice switched to TVS with Doppler blood flow imaging as it is superior to the transabdominal approach. In TVS, the probe is near the ovary with no airspace as in transabdominal approach.

The United Kingdom Collaborative Trial of Ovarian Cancer Screening (UKCTOCS) addressed the effect of screening on mortality. The trial recruited postmenopausal women (50–74 years). The participants were assigned to control, multimodal screening (MMS) using CA125 with TVS as a second line test, and the third group underwent annual TVS (USS). The results reported include surgical intervention rate, which was similar in MMS and USS groups. A similar number of primary ovarian and tubal cancers were detected. The invasive cancers detected were stage I/II, which is reasonably early detection. Comparison of the PPV, sensitivity, and specificity of the two modalities demonstrated a statistically significant difference in specificity only [21].

Classification of ovarian morphology adopted in UKCTOCS normal morphology, simple cyst, and complex morphology. Simple cyst criteria include a single, thin-walled cyst with no septa or papillae. A complex cyst is one not fitting with simple cyst criteria. The normal category is normal ovarian dimensions. The pelvic sonography features that were recoded for statistical analysis included the number and size of cysts, wall regularity, presence and thickness of septae, size of papillae, and echogenicity of fluid contents. Classification of cysts and complex morphology was based on International Ovarian Tumor Analysis (IOTA) classification. This classification categorizes cysts on different scales named B and M, given numerical values with the letter. Visualization of the ovaries was confirmed by objective measurement of the ovary and calculating its volume using the formula (d1xd2xd3x0.532). Inability to visualize the ovary should be supported by obtaining a good view of iliac vessels. Poor view due to obstruction by the bowel, fibroids, pelvic varicosities, or for other reasons needs to be documented. Ascites was defined as a maximum vertical pool measurement of greater than or equal to 10 mm. Cysts up to 60 $cm^3$ are considered within normal ovarian morphology. Abnormal ovarian morphology includes ascites, complex morphology, or cysts larger than 60 $cm^3$ [21].

Complex morphology and ovarian cysts are assessed using IOTA classification based on B and M features. B stands for predicting benign conditions, while M stands for predicting malignancy. The M is classified into five groups, from M1 to M5. The same applies to the B group, from B1 to B5. The structural descriptions include echogenic consistency, complexity, ascites, wall regularity, septation, papillae, and blood flow. These sonographic findings are grouped for risk scoring to predict the possibility of cancer prior to surgical intervention [22].

Sonographic features suggestive of cancer in an ultrasound score in the Risk of Malignancy Index (RMI) include multilocularity, solid areas, bilateral masses, and evidence of metastasis [16].

The Ovarian Morphology Index (OMI) is based on three structural components:

- Ovarian Volume ranging from 10 to 500 $cm^3$ (0–4 score).
- Wall structure is either smooth or with papillary projections with a cutoff thickness of 3 mm.
- Septal structure ranging from no septa, thin septa, thick septa, and solid mass.

OMI was developed at the University of Kentucky for use in the Ovarian Cancer Screening Project. A score of 0–4 was assigned for each of the three structural components. Statistical evaluation of OMI scores revealed a sensitivity of 89% and a positive predictive value of 46%. The use of OMI is an effective and cost-efficient method of increasing the positive predictive value of TVS screening for ovarian cancer [23].

The PLCO trial recruited 78,216 participants (55–74 years old) over the period from November 1993 to July 2001. Participants were randomized to the annual screening group (39105) and usual care group (39111). The main outcome measure was mortality from ovarian cancer. The intervention group was subjected to annual screening with CA125 for 6 years and TVS for 4 years. Participants were followed for 13 years. The screening program did not reduce ovarian cancer mortality. Moreover, out of the 3285 who tested false positive, 1080 underwent surgical follow-up, of whom 163 (15%) experienced at least one serious complication [24].

The Shizuoka Cohort Study of Ovarian Cancer Screening (SCSOCS) randomized control trial recruited 41,688 (intervention group) and 40,799 (control group) participants during 1985–1999 with a follow-up mean of 9.2 years. The interventions offered were sequential ultrasound and serum CA125 measurement. With successive screenings, the detection rate increased. Detection of early disease stage I ovarian cancer was higher in the screen group compared to the control group; however, the difference did not reach statistical significance [25].

Pelvic sonography as a screening tool for ovarian cancer in the general population has statistical values and criteria different from those in women with pelvic masses. There is room for improvement in the detection rate and characterization of pathological findings with the development of machine resolution, use of 3D and 4D machines, contrast-enhanced ultrasound, application of artificial intelligence (AI) and machine learning to improve interpretation, and elastography to assess tissue stiffness. Pelvic sonography is more likely to be utilized as a secondary screening tool. Cases picked with primary tools that are not expensive, feasible, or do not need skilled personnel can be screened with pelvic sonography.

### 4.4 High-risk population screening

The concept of screening in a normal population is different from a high-risk population. Women at high risk of ovarian cancer by virtue of known predisposing germ line mutation or strong family history of ovarian or other associated cancers are at increased risk of developing ovarian cancer as well as other types of cancers. This category is offered prophylactic salpingoophorectomy as a risk-reducing intervention.

This intervention will reduce the risk of primary ovarian cancer by up to 80%. Since the risk is not eliminated, the need for screening persists. This risk-reducing "not preventive" procedure when carried out in premenopausal women is associated with the health hazards of surgical menopause. Delaying the procedure after menopause makes the need for ovarian cancer screening justified. Unlike bilateral salpingo-oophorectomy, it has been hoped that screening may permit detection at a point in the disease's natural history where cure is still possible. The UK Familial Ovarian Cancer Screening Study (UKFOCSS) recruited more than 5000 women at high risk of ovarian cancer between 2002 and 2009 [26].

### 4.5 Cost-effectiveness analysis

Cost-Effectiveness of Screening postmenopausal women in the UK using multimodal screening (MMS) in UKCTOCS published by Kearns et al. demonstrated that screening for ovarian cancer with MMS is both more effective and more expensive than not screening [27]. MMS was more costly but more effective, with an incremental cost-effectiveness ratio (ICER) of £8864 per quality adjusted life year (QALY). Adopting a two-step screening model with annual CA125, if tested positive, pelvic sonography is performed, yielding an ICER of $88,993 per year of life saved. The estimated mortality reduction is 13%. The expected detection rate of stage I disease is 34%, compared to 18% in no screening model [28].

### 4.6 Symptom-based screening

Retrospective analysis of symptoms associated significantly with epithelial ovarian cancer has been suggested as a potential tool for symptom-based screening. The symptoms to be addressed include:

- Pelvic/abdominal pain, which is dull aching of chronic nature.
- Urinary urgency/frequency is the least important symptom related to the development of epithelial ovarian cancer.
- Increased abdominal size/bloating due to gaseous distension or ascites.
- Difficulty eating/feeling full as part of fullness of loss of appetite.

These symptoms are present for less than a year and occur more than 12 days per month.

A total of 149 women with confirmed epithelial ovarian cancer completed a survey of the above symptoms. A case-control study compared symptoms type, frequency, severity, and duration between confirmatory and exploratory groups. Statistical analysis using a logistic regression model confirmed the significance of abdominal-pelvic pain, increased abdominal size with or without bloating, and difficulty eating with a feeling of fullness as possible predictors of the diagnosis of ovarian cancer. A symptoms index (SI) was considered positive if any of these six symptoms occurred more than 12 days per month for less than 1 year.

The sensitivity of SI ranges from 56.7% in early disease to 79.5% for advanced disease. The specificity of SI is affected by age. Depression was significantly more common in women who had cancer compared with other groups. Evaluation of the symptoms index in the general population at a primary care clinic revealed that 2.6% of participants tested positive. Compared to CA125, the statistical values of SI are almost similar for different disease stages. The cost of symptom index is less compared to CA125 measurement [29]. Retrospective studies of women with ovarian cancer documented missed opportunities if SI was adopted. Prior to the confirmed diagnosis of ovarian cancer, women are more likely to have visits the above symptoms to health facilities [30].

Ovarian cancer being nominated as a silent killer due to late presentation. Delay in diagnosis has been attributed in part to physicians and health care providers. Women with a significant symptom index are directed to primary care, not to gynecology departments. Moreover, screening with these symptoms is not technically feasible in view of the busy primary care clinics. Use of artificial intelligence programs may prove to be valuable, as a scoring system for index symptoms may detect women who are candidates for diagnostic testing.

A retrospective study of SI in women with high-risk early-stage ovarian cancer enrolled in a clinical trial showed that more than 70% of patients with high-risk early-stage epithelial ovarian cancer presented with one or more symptoms before the confirmation of cancer diagnosis. The most common being abdominal/pelvic pain. The analysis of results confirmed a relationship between tumor size and symptom index frequency [31].

Using shopping data to improve the diagnosis of ovarian cancer was studied using computational analysis of a web-based survey. Key knowledge about health care purchases collected by a web-based survey was analyzed to link purchases to symptoms related to presentation to health care and timing of diagnosis. The analysis of the web-based survey showed the potential predictive value of shopping purchases. Analysis addressed the role of health care provider advice, which did not address the possibility of ovarian cancer as a potential cause for the symptoms-related purchases. The purchases were directed by the health care provider. The findings are consistent with the symptom index model, as the shopping data target abdominal pain symptoms in the majority of cases. Women's shopping data could be potentially useful for early ovarian cancer detection [32].

Symptom-based ovarian cancer screening using the modified Goff Symptom Index (GSI) was tested in a case-control study in an Indian population. The sensitivity of modified GSI was 71.6%. The addition of two symptoms (loss of appetite and weight) improved the sensitivity to 77% without compromising specificity (88.5%). The modified GSI addresses 10 symptoms given a scale of 1–5 according to presence, severity, frequency, and duration. The symptom index is considered positive for ovarian cancer screening if the frequency of symptoms is at least 12 times per month for less than 1 year. Analysis of symptom cluster did not prove statistical significance of increased urinary frequency/urgency. This is not the case for abdominal/pelvic pain, bloating/increased abdominal size, and difficulty in eating/feeling full. These symptoms proved to be statistically significant when tested in a case-control study. Validation of urinary symptoms may be required before incorporation in a symptom-based screening model. Symptom-based screening suggested by Goff included six symptoms. All were gastrointestinal. This could explain the reason behind the delay in initiating measures to reach the diagnosis. The patient will seek advice from a specialist other than a gynecologist, whose ovary is out of his scope of thinking as the reason behind the gastrointestinal symptoms. The six symptoms were clustered into three groups. Urinary symptoms were suggested later by Kim upon validation of GSI in a Korean population [33, 34]. Screening ovarian cancer with a symptoms index is a promising model with a fascinating future in the coming era of artificial intelligence (AI). Friendly software to be used by women can be implemented. This will improve efficacy and reduce costs, in addition to reducing the utilization of health facilities. Validation of symptom index screening in different populations is challenging. The criteria need to be scrutinized and validated to achieve the maximum sensitivity without compromising specificity.

Combining the symptoms index with CA125 as predictors of ovarian cancer improved the sensitivity from 65.5 to 85.3% at the expense of a specificity drop to 59.5%. Positive predictive value may increase with the addition of TVS as a secondary tool for screening [34].

The sensitivity and specificity of the symptoms index vary with stage of ovarian cancer and age of women. The sensitivity of the symptom index for stage I/II disease is 44.8%, compared to 72.9% for stage III/IV. In the case of adopting 50 years as a cutoff, sensitivity and specificity vary with age. Before the age of 50 years, a sensitivity of 81.9% was reported for a specificity of 58.5%. Women above 50 years demonstrated a sensitivity of 69.3% for a specificity of 89% [34].

### 4.7 MicroRNAs

MicroRNAs such as miR-200 and miR-214 are potential biomarkers for ovarian cancer. Detection and pattern may give valuable information about ovarian cancer and the progression of the disease. MicroRNAs, being noncoding RNAs, are involved in carcinogenesis as well as other aspects of cellular mechanisms such as cell cycle, apoptosis, proliferation, invasion, and metastasis. MicroRNAs may play a potential therapeutic role. MicroRNAs regulate 60% of human genes. MicroRNAs can be upregulated or downregulated with different impacts on oncogenesis. There is emerging evidence that circulating microRNAs, unlike cellular forms, are stable as they are not degraded by the RNase enzyme [35].

### 4.8 Proteomes

Multiple studies reported characterization of biomarkers that may potentially prove effective screening tools. Monocyte chemoattractant protein-1 (MCP-1) and Interleucin-8 (IL-8) obtained from ovarian fluid cysts significantly correlate with ovarian malignancy [36].

Urinary micro-peptides characterized in women with ovarian cancer include catalase, α1 acid glycoprotein, and peroxiredoxin. These urinary micro-peptides prove a significance correlation higher than CA125 [37].

Intrauterine lavage (IUL) has been studied based on the concept of tubal origin of ovarian cancer. The tubal cells may be detected by uterine washings as the malignant cell may travel down. The levels of CA125 and HE4 in IUL were measured. The concept in this modality is to assess tissue biomarkers, not serum levels. Results are promising as the. IUL has detected mutations in TP53 as well [38].

The potential role of circulating DNA (ctDNA) is promising. Invasive tumors release mutant DNA in the circulation. Testing for ctDNA may improve the sensitivity of ovarian cancer screening [39].

Contrast-enhanced TVS has been suggested as a tool that will improve detection of neovascularity in the ovary. This can be incorporated in the TVS arm as a screening tool. Detection of neovascularity may help discriminate benign from possible malignant ovarian neoplasm [40].

*DOI: http://dx.doi.org/10.5772/intechopen.1007912*

## 5. Conclusion

Ovarian cancer screening is not currently recommended. This recommendation is based on the statistical characteristics of the screening tests available. There is an overwhelming need for a successful ovarian cancer screening program, as ovarian cancer is the second leading cause of malignancy in women. The obstacles include the anatomical site of the ovary, the lack of precursor lesions, the low positive predictive value of screening tools, the significant hazards of interventions based on screening results currently practiced, and the lack of positive impact on mortality with the screening tools currently available. There are great potentials for future developments using AI, circulating DNA, mRNA, proteoms, and micro-peptides that may yield sound statistical value with successful cost-effective and safe ovarian cancer screening that improves quality of life and reduces mortality.

## Conflict of interest

The author declares no conflict of interest.

## Author details

Abubakr Mohamed Ali Nasr[1,2]

1 Department of Obstetrician and Gynaecologist, National Gurad Health Affairs, Prince Mohamed Bin Abdelaziz Hospital, Kingdom of Saudi Arabia

2 Faculty of Medicine, University of Khartoum, Sudan

*Address all correspondence to: abubakrnasr@gmail.com

## References

[1] Cuckle H. Principles of screening. The Obstetrician & Gynaecologist. RCOG. USA: Wiley Online Library; 2004. pp. 6:1-6:22. DOI: 10.1576/ toag.6.1.21.26976

[2] US Preventive Services Task Force, Grossman DC, Curry SJ, Owens DK, Barry MJ, Davidson KW, et al. Screening for ovarian cancer: US preventive services task force recommendation statement. Journal of the American Medical Association. 2018;**319**(6):588-594. DOI: 10.1001/jama.2017.21926

[3] Clarke-Pearson DL. Clinical practice. Screening for ovarian cancer. The New England Journal of Medicine. 2009;**361**(2):170-177. DOI: 10.1056/NEJMcp0901926

[4] Fathalla MF. Incessant ovulation—A factor in ovarian neoplasia? The Lancet [Internet]. 1971;**298**(7716):163. DOI: 10.1016/s0140-6736(71)92335-x

[5] Fathalla MF. Incessant ovulation and ovarian cancer - a hypothesis re-visited. Facts, Views & Vision in ObGyn. 2013;**5**(4):292-297

[6] Feeney L, Harley IJ, McCluggage WG, Mullan PB, Beirne JP. Liquid biopsy in ovarian cancer: Catching the silent killer before it strikes. World Journal of Clinical Oncology. 2020;**11**(11):868-889. DOI: 10.5306/wjco.v11.i11.868

[7] Kurman RJ, Visvanathan K, Roden R, Wu TC, IeM S. Early detection and treatment of ovarian cancer: Shifting from early stage to minimal volume of disease based on a new model of carcinogenesis. American Journal of Obstetrics and Gynecology. 2008;**198**(4):351-356. DOI: 10.1016/j.ajog.2008.01.005

[8] Finch A, Beiner M, Lubinski J, Lynch HT, Moller P, Rosen B, et al. Hereditary ovarian cancer clinical study group. Salpingo-oophorectomy and the risk of ovarian, fallopian tube, and peritoneal cancers in women with a BRCA1 or BRCA2 mutation. Journal of the American Medical Association. 2006;**296**(2):185-192. DOI: 10.1001/jama.296.2.185

[9] Piek JM, van Diest PJ, Zweemer RP, Jansen JW, Poort-Keesom RJ, Menko FH, et al. Dysplastic changes in prophylactically removed fallopian tubes of women predisposed to developing ovarian cancer. The Journal of Pathology. 2001;**195**(4):451-456. DOI: 10.1002/path.1000

[10] Kindelberger DW, Lee Y, Miron A, Hirsch MS, Feltmate C, Medeiros F, et al. Intraepithelial carcinoma of the fimbria and pelvic serous carcinoma: Evidence for a causal relationship. The American Journal of Surgical Pathology. 2007;**31**(2):161-169. DOI: 10.1097/01.pas.0000213335.40358.47

[11] Bast RC Jr, Feeney M, Lazarus H, Nadler LM, Colvin RB, Knapp RC. Reactivity of a monoclonal antibody with human ovarian carcinoma. The Journal of Clinical Investigation. 1981;**68**(5):1331-1337. DOI: 10.1172/jci110380

[12] Jacobs I, Bast RC Jr. The CA 125 tumour-associated antigen: A review of the literature. Human Reproduction. 1989;**4**(1):1-12. DOI: 10.1093/oxfordjournals.humrep.a136832

[13] Kabawat SE, Bast RC Jr, Bhan AK, Welch WR, Knapp RC, Colvin RB. Tissue distribution of a coelomic-epithelium-related antigen recognized by the monoclonal antibody OC125. International Journal of Gynecological

Pathology. 1983;**2**(3):275-285. DOI: 10.1097/00004347-198303000-00005

[14] Cramer DW, Bast RC Jr, Berg CD, Diamandis EP, Godwin AK, Hartge P, et al. Ovarian cancer biomarker performance in prostate, lung, colorectal, and ovarian cancer screening trial specimens. Cancer Prevention Research (Philadelphia, PA.). 2011;**4**(3):365-374. DOI: 10.1158/1940-6207.CAPR-10-0195

[15] Moore RG, McMeekin DS, Brown AK, DiSilvestro P, Miller MC, Allard WJ, et al. A novel multiple marker bioassay utilizing HE4 and CA125 for the prediction of ovarian cancer in patients with a pelvic mass. Gynecologic Oncology. 2009;**112**(1):40-46. DOI: 10.1016/j.ygyno.2008.08.031. Epub 2008 Oct 12

[16] Jacobs I, Oram D, Fairbanks J, Turner J, Frost C, Grudzinskas JG. A risk of malignancy index incorporating CA 125, ultrasound and menopausal status for the accurate preoperative diagnosis of ovarian cancer. British Journal of Obstetrics and Gynaecology. 1990;**97**(10):922-929. DOI: 10.1111/j.1471-0528.1990.tb02448.x

[17] Bailey J, Tailor A, Naik R, Lopes A, Godfrey K, Hatem HM, et al. Risk of malignancy index for referral of ovarian cancer cases to a tertiary center: Does it identify the correct cases? International Journal of Gynecological Cancer. 2006;**16**(Suppl. 1):30-34. DOI: 10.1111/j.1525-1438.2006.00468.x

[18] Skates SJ, Menon U, MacDonald N, Rosenthal AN, Oram DH, Knapp RC, et al. Calculation of the risk of ovarian cancer from serial CA-125 values for preclinical detection in postmenopausal women. Journal of Clinical Oncology. 2003;**21**(Suppl. 10):206s-210s. DOI: 10.1200/JCO.2003.02.955

[19] Heilbrun ME, Olpin J, Shaaban A. Imaging of benign adnexal masses: Characteristic presentations on ultrasound, computed tomography, and magnetic resonance imaging. Clinical Obstetrics and Gynecology. 2009;**52**(1):21-39. DOI: 10.1097/GRF.0b013e318195834b

[20] Campbell S, Bhan V, Royston P, Whitehead MI, Collins WP. Transabdominal ultrasound screening for early ovarian cancer. BMJ. 1989;**299**(6712):1363-1367. DOI: 10.1136/bmj.299.6712.1363

[21] Menon U, Gentry-Maharaj A, Hallett R, Ryan A, Burnell M, Sharma A, et al. Sensitivity and specificity of multimodal and ultrasound screening for ovarian cancer, and stage distribution of detected cancers: Results of the prevalence screen of the UK collaborative trial of ovarian cancer screening (UKCTOCS). The Lancet Oncology. 2009;**10**(4):327-340. DOI: 10.1016/S1470-2045(09)70026-9. Epub 2009 Mar 11

[22] Timmerman D, Ameye L, Fischerova D, Epstein E, Melis GB, Guerriero S, et al. Simple ultrasound rules to distinguish between benign and malignant adnexal masses before surgery: Prospective validation by IOTA group. BMJ. 2010;**341**:c6839. DOI: 10.1136/bmj.c6839

[23] DePriest PD, Varner E, Powell J, Fried A, Puls L, Higgins R, et al. The efficacy of a sonographic morphology index in identifying ovarian cancer: A multi-institutional investigation. Gynecologic Oncology. 1994;**55**(2):174-178. DOI: 10.1006/gyno.1994.1273

[24] Buys SS, Partridge E, Black A, Johnson CC, Lamerato L, Isaacs C, et al. Effect of screening on ovarian cancer mortality: The prostate, lung, colorectal

and ovarian (PLCO) cancer screening randomized controlled trial. JAMA. 2011;**305**(22):2295-2303. DOI: 10.1001/jama.2011.766

[25] Kobayashi H, Yamada Y, Sado T, Sakata M, Yoshida S, Kawaguchi R, et al. A randomized study of screening for ovarian cancer: A multicenter study in Japan. International Journal of Gynecological Cancer. 2008;**18**(3):414-420. DOI: 10.1111/j.1525-1438.2007.01035.x. Epub 2007 Jul 21

[26] Rosenthal AN. Ovarian cancer screening in the high-risk population--the UK familial ovarian cancer screening study (UKFOCSS). International Journal of Gynecological Cancer. 2012;**22**(Suppl. 1):S27-S28. DOI: 10.1097/IGC.0b013e318251cc3f

[27] Kearns B, Chilcott J, Whyte S, Preston L, Sadler S. Cost-effectiveness of screening for ovarian cancer amongst postmenopausal women: A model-based economic evaluation. BMC Medicine. 2016;**14**(1):200. DOI: 10.1186/s12916-016-0743-y. Erratum in: BMC Med. 2017;15(1):31, 10.1186/s12916-017-0803-y

[28] Kwon JS. Cost-effectiveness of ovarian cancer prevention strategies. Clinical Obstetrics and Gynecology. 2017;**60**(4):780-788. DOI: 10.1097/GRF.0000000000000317

[29] Goff BA, Mandel LS, Drescher CW, Urban N, Gough S, Schurman KM, et al. Development of an ovarian cancer symptom index: Possibilities for earlier detection. Cancer. 2007;**109**(2):221-227. DOI: 10.1002/cncr.22371

[30] Smith LH, Morris CR, Yasmeen S, Parikh-Patel A, Cress RD, Romano PS. Ovarian cancer: Can we make the clinical diagnosis earlier? Cancer. 2005;**104**(7):1398-1407. DOI: 10.1002/cncr.21310

[31] Chan JK, Tian C, Kesterson JP, Monk BJ, Kapp DS, Davidson B, et al. Symptoms of women with high-risk early-stage ovarian cancer. Obstetrics and Gynecology. 2022;**139**(2):157-162. DOI: 10.1097/AOG.0000000000004642

[32] Dolan EH, Goulding J, Tata LJ, Lang AR. Using shopping data to improve the diagnosis of ovarian cancer: Computational analysis of a web-based survey. JMIR Cancer. 2023;**9**:e37141. DOI: 10.2196/37141

[33] Shetty J, Priyadarshini P, Pandey D, Manjunath AP. Modified Goff symptom index: Simple triage tool for ovarian malignancy. Sultan Qaboos University Medical Journal. 2015;**15**(3):e370-e375. DOI: 10.18295/squmj.2015.15.03.011 Epub 2015 Aug 24

[34] Kim MK, Kim K, Kim SM, Kim JW, Park NH, Song YS, et al. A hospital-based case-control study of identifying ovarian cancer using symptom index. Journal of Gynecologic Oncology. 2009;**20**(4):238-242. DOI: 10.3802/jgo.2009.20.4.238 Epub 2009 Dec 28

[35] Kinose Y, Sawada K, Nakamura K, Kimura T. The role of microRNAs in ovarian cancer. BioMed Research International. 2014;**2014**:249393. DOI: 10.1155/2014/249393. Epub 2014 Sep 10

[36] Kristjánsdóttir B, Partheen K, Fung ET, Yip C, Levan K, Sundfeldt K. Early inflammatory response in epithelial ovarian tumor cyst fluids. Cancer Medicine. 2014;**3**(5):1302-1312. DOI: 10.1002/cam4.282. Epub 2014 Jun 20

[37] Murgan SS, Abd Elaziz FJ, Nasr AMA, Elfaki MEE, Khalil EAG. Ovarian cancer: Tumor-specific urinary micro-peptides profiling as potential biomarkers for early diagnosis.

Proteomes. 2020;**8**(4):32. DOI: 10.3390/proteomes8040032

[38] Sia TY, Yaari Z, Feiner R, Smith E, Da Cruz PA, Selenica P, et al. Uterine washings as a novel method for early detection of ovarian cancer: Trials and tribulations. Gynecologic Oncology Reports. 2024;**51**:101330. DOI: 10.1016/j.gore.2024.101330

[39] Prasanth BK, Alkhowaiter S, Sawarkar G, Dharshini BD, Baskaran R, A. Unlocking early cancer detection: Exploring biomarkers, circulating DNA, and innovative technological approaches. Cureus. 2023;**15**(12):e51090. DOI: 10.7759/cureus.51090

[40] van Nagell JR, Jr HJT. Transvaginal ultrasonography in ovarian cancer screening: Current perspectives. International Journal of Women's Health. 2013;**6**:25-33. DOI: 10.2147/IJWH.S38347

Chapter 3

# Molecular Characterization of Endometrial Cancers and Therapeutic Implications

*Tamara Kalir*

## Abstract

Endometrial cancer is the most common uterine malignancy in the U.S. and Europe; a significant cause of morbidity and mortality in these countries. Endometrial cancer historically was classified into two groups, termed Type I and Type II as described by JV Bokhman in 1983. Over time, it was recognized that a major challenge existed in the realm of histopathologic diagnosis of endometrial cancers. While there was good agreement among pathologists in the diagnosis of low-grade (well and moderately differentiated) endometrial carcinomas, the same could not be said for all high-grade tumors. In 2013 a new, 4-tier molecular classification scheme for the pathologic diagnosis of endometrial cancer was proposed by DA Levine and The Cancer Genome Atlas Research Network, and this scheme has had ground-breaking implications. The then-newly proposed scheme has been validated by various investigators and has resulted in a revised, 2023 FIGO staging for endometrial cancers. The 4-tier scheme has enabled: (i) better prognostication, (ii) improved reproducibility in the pathologic diagnosis of high-grade endometrial cancers, (iii) improved stratification of patients for targeted therapy and clinical trials, (iv) better patient management, i.e., less over- and under-treatments administered, and (v) identification of women at greater risk for having Lynch syndrome.

**Keywords:** molecular, serous, endometrioid, carcinoma, p53, mutation, DNA, mismatch, repair, deficiency, FIGO, 2023, stage, immunotherapy, target, HER2

## 1. Introduction

Endometrial cancer is the most common uterine corpus malignancy in the United States and Europe. The American Cancer Society [1] estimates for the year 2024 endometrial cancer will afflict 67,880 women and cause 13,250 deaths. Medical scientists are continuing their search for better ways to help endometrial cancer patients. Management of endometrial cancer has long relied on the histopathologic diagnosis, as this has contributed both to endometrial cancer staging as well as played a role in post-operative management. Hence the importance of histopathological classification of this cancer. The classification of endometrial cancer has in the past been based on a dualistic model, as published in a landmark paper by JV Bokhman in 1983. In his paper, Bokhman [2] detailed the characteristics of his studies of 366 patients over a period of 20 years, from which he concluded that there are two main types of endometrial carcinomas, which he termed Type I and Type II. The Type I cancers comprised roughly 65% of all endometrial cancers in his study group. Type I cancers appeared to be estrogen-driven, typically occurring in obese, nulliparous patients who may have had other elements of metabolic syndrome such as hypercholesterolemia, diabetes and hypertension. Endometrial hyperplasia was common in these women. Almost 80% of the patients in this group had low grade (FIGO G1 or G2) cancers while only 20% had high grade (G3) tumors. In contrast, the type II cancer patients comprised roughly 35% of all endometrial cancer cases in his study. These patients lacked metabolic syndrome and tended to have high grade tumors in 65.7% of cases. The type II tumors tended to be deeply invasive into the myometrium compared to a minority of type I tumors (only 30.4% in his study). Pelvic lymph node metastases were significantly more prevalent in type II cancers as compared with type I tumors (27.8 versus 9.4%). Women with type I tumors had better 5 year survival (85.6%) compared with those in the type II group (58.8%); for which metastases and recurrence occurred within the first few years following treatment.

Subsequent series studies supported Bokhman's clinical associations. Wang et al. [3] compared risk factors, prognosis and clinical factors for type I and II endometrial cancers in 606 patients. They found that compared with type I cases, the type II cancer patients tended to be older, their cancers were higher stage, associated with greater incidence of myometrial invasion, cervical involvement and metastases to lymph nodes, with poorer overall survival and progression free survival. And stimulated by Bokhman's work, other authors searched to better understand the pathogenesis of endometrial cancers. In 1995 Sherman et al. [4] postulated that, based on the differences in the clinical, histologic and prognostic features of the type I and II carcinomas, the pathogenesis of these tumors should also differ. To test their hypothesis, they performed immunohistochemical studies on the expression of p53 protein in ninety-five specimens, including forty-eight hysterectomies and forty-seven endometrial biopsy samples, which encompassed 45 endometrioid carcinomas, 28 serous carcinomas, 10 carcinosarcomas, 6 mixed endometrioid/serous carcinomas, and 2 clear cell carcinomas. Eight cases exhibited endometrial hyperplasia in association with endometrioid carcinoma. Twenty eight cases exhibited intraepithelial carcinoma; most of these in association with serous carcinoma. On the basis of p53 immunostaining, they were able to stratify the endometrial cancers into cases that did not exhibit abnormal p53 expression, and cases that did exhibit p53 abnormal expression (mostly overexpression but some cases with absent expression). Putative precursor lesions (endometrial hyperplasia and endometrial intraepithelial carcinoma, respectively) showed similar staining to their invasive endometrioid adenocarcinoma and serous carcinoma counterparts. Benign endometrial samples and atypical endometrial hyperplasia samples were nonreactive as were 80% of endometrioid carcinomas. In eighty-six percent of serous carcinomas containing endometrial intraepithelial carcinoma (EIC), both components showed abnormal p53 expression. Immunoreactivity for p53 was also found in 100% of clear cell carcinomas, 83% of mixed endometrioid/serous carcinomas, and 70% of carcinosarcomas. On the basis of these findings, the authors were able to stratify endometrial cancers into two groups: the endometrial hyperplasia – endometrioid carcinoma group which generally tended not to exhibit p53 overexpression, and the endometrial intraepithelial carcinoma (EIC)/serous carcinoma groups which tended to show p53 overexpression. They postulated that a p53 mutational pathway was unrelated to the estrogen-stimulated hyperplasia/carcinoma pathway; in support of the dualistic model of endometrial carcinogenesis. The hyperplasia-to-cancer hypothesis was supported in 2003 when Lukanova et al. [5], performed a multicenter, international prospective, case-control study of 124 postmenopausal women with endometrial cancer. They measured pre-diagnostic blood concentrations of androstenedione, estrone, estradiol, testosterone, sex hormone binding globulin and dehydroepiandrosterone. Two controls per case were matched for age and recruitment date. Patients using hormone replacement therapy were excluded. The authors found a strong and direct association between circulating sex steroid hormones with endometrial cancer, and an inverse association of sex hormone binding globulin levels. They felt that the androstenedione and testosterone effects were mediated via their conversion to estrogens. These and other studies supported the dualistic categorization of endometrial cancer; with endometrioid carcinomas and serous carcinomas comprising the most common histotypes of Bokhman's type I and type II carcinomas, respectively.

## 2. Problems in the pathologic diagnosis of endometrial cancers

A major challenge existed in the realm of histopathologic categorization of endometrial cancers. While there was good agreement among pathologists in the diagnosis of low-grade (well and moderately differentiated) endometrial carcinomas, the same could not be said for all high-grade tumors. **Figures 1** and **2** illustrate the similarity of two high-grade endometrial cancers of different histotype, for demonstration purposes. While architecturally similar, a very subtle difference between the tumors can be seen in the presence of ever-so-slightly larger, somewhat more eosinophilic nucleoli in the serous carcinoma (**Figure 1**) compared to the slightly smaller, more basophilic nucleoli in the endometrioid carcinoma (**Figure 2**). In their 2013 study, Gilks et al. [6] collected fifty-six cases of high-grade endometrial carcinoma from the Vancouver General Hospital surgical pathology archives. Each case was reviewed in its entirety by three pathologists who independently diagnosed subtype and in the case of mixed carcinomas, designated a percentage of each subtype. They found that all three reviewers

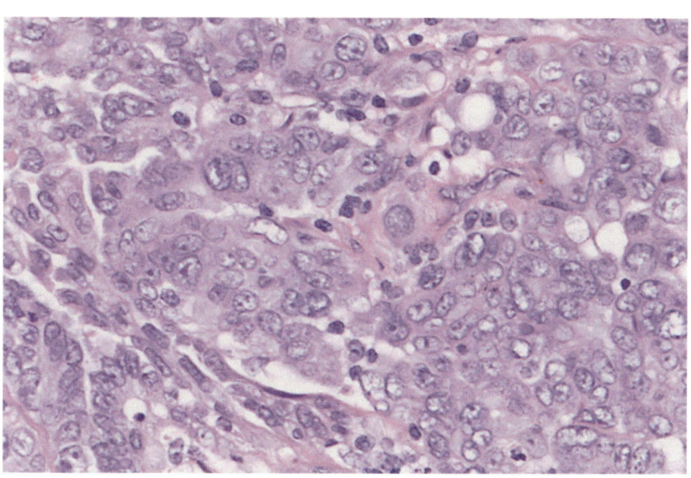

**Figure 1.**
*Serous carcinoma, hematoxylin-and-eosin stain.*

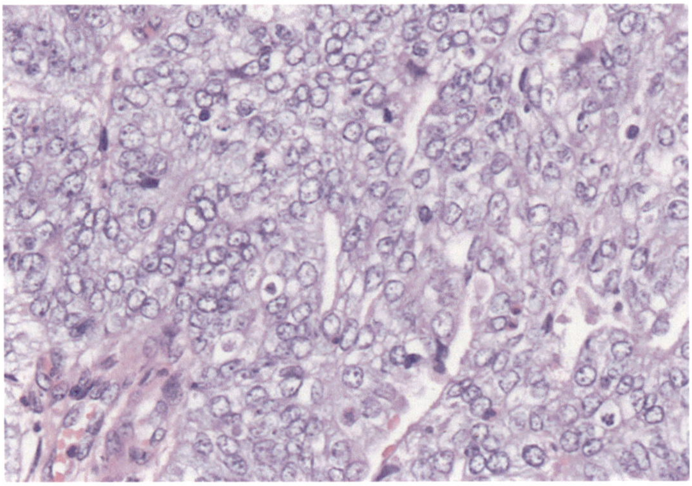

**Figure 2.**
*Endometrioid carcinoma, hematoxylin-and-eosin stain.*

agreed in 62.5%, or 35 of the 56 cases; specifically of the subtype in pure cases and the major high-grade subtype in mixed tumors. The reviewers had major disagreement in seventeen of the fifty six, or 35.8% of the cases and, in 17 of these cases (30.4%) there was no consensus about the major subtype diagnosis. In an additional fraction of cases, there was minor disagreement about the minor high-grade component subtype in a mixed tumor in 4 of the 56 cases, or 7.1% of cases. In 3, or 5.4% of cases, there was disagreement about whether a component of high-grade endometrial carcinoma was present. The most common areas for disagreement were serous or clear cell carcinoma (7 cases), and serous or high-grade (grade 3) endometrioid carcinoma (6 cases). For the cases in which there was disagreement about whether the tumor was serous or endometrioid, a 5-marker immunohistochemical panel was constructed for markers: p16, PTEN, p53, ER and PR, for purposes of adjudication. For the six disagreed-upon cases of serous versus high-grade endometrioid carcinoma, the immuno-panel showed that four of the cases were serous carcinomas and two of the cases were endometrioid carcinomas. The authors also conducted pairwise comparisons between reviewers for the 20 cases which showed major disagreement. They found that paired reviewers (comparing reviewers 1 and 2, comparing reviewers 2 and 3, and comparing reviewers 1 and 3) showed agreements in respectively: 5/20, cases, 8/20 cases, and 7/20 cases. These roughly similar numbers suggested that disagreement was not likely to be a result of systematic bias on any one reviewer's part (i.e., a result of a single reviewer having outlier opinions). Overall the authors concluded that there was rather poor reproducibility among pathologists in diagnosing high-grade endometrial carcinoma subtypes, and utilization of molecular tools would aid in accuracy and reproducibility in the diagnosis.

## 3. Molecular classification of endometrial cancers

Concurrently or perhaps serendipitously in 2013, a proposal for a new molecular classification scheme for endometrial cancer was published by DA Levine & The Cancer Genome Atlas (TCGA) Research Network [7], stratifying endometrial cancers into four groups, rather than the historical two groups, based on their study of 373 endometrial cancers. Using microarray- and sequencing-based technologies for genomic, transcriptomic and proteomic analysis, they identified four molecular categories: (i) tumors which harbored pathogenic mutations in the exonuclease domain of the polymerase-epsilon (POL-e) gene, designated as POLE-ultramutated, (ii) microsatellite instability hypermutated tumors, most of which exhibited MLH1 promoter methylation, (iii) tumors that were mostly microsatellite stable and showed low mutational frequency, designated as no specific molecular profile (NSMP), and (iv) tumors which harbored pathogenic mutations in the TP53 gene and also showed extensive somatic copy number alterations. There were some correlations of the molecular groups with the histologic groups. For example, microsatellite instability was seen in 40% of their endometrioid (type I) tumors and only 2% of serous (type II) tumors, and serous-like tumors had fewer PTEN mutations (11%) compared to endometrioid tumors (84%). They found that tumors in the serous-like group had worse progression-free survival compared with tumors in the endometrioid groups. However, the groups did not correlate completely with histologic types in that serous tumors, mixed carcinoma tumors and 12% of their endometrioid tumors which included 24% grade 3 and 5% grade 1 or 2 tumors, clustered into the fourth (serous-like) group. Tumors in this group also exhibited amplifications in MYC, ERBB2 and CCNE1 oncogenes and FGFR3 and SX17 in addition to frequent TP53 mutations. The POLE ultramutated group showed an increased Cytosine-to-Adenine transversion frequency occurring in the exonuclease domain of the gene. POLE, referring to the catalytic subunit of DNA polymerase epsilon, is important in DNA replication and repair. They found hotspot mutations at Pro286Arg and Val411.Leu in 76% of the ultramutated samples. Other genes which were mutated in this subset included: PTEN, PIK3R1, PIK3CA, KRAS and FBXW7. POLE ultramutated tumors showed the best progression-free survival among the four groups; the TP53 mutated group exhibited the worst prognosis, and the other two groups showed intermediate prognosis. In the microsatellite instability group, tumors showed roughly tenfold greater mutational frequency than the microsatellite stable endometrioid carcinomas, few somatic copy number alterations, KRAS mutations, and a few mutations in FBXW7, CTNNB1, PPP2R1A and TP53. In the microsatellite stable group, authors found a high frequency of CTNNB1 mutations (52%). In one case, a serous carcinoma was found to lack TP53 mutation and extensive somatic copy number alterations, and had a KRAS mutation. Upon re-review of the histological section, this case was re-classified as a grade 3 endometrioid tumor, demonstrating how molecular testing may be helpful in tumoral classification and thereby significantly impact decisions regarding treatment.

Because the TCGA classification lacked the statistical power to prove clinical relevance, other groups worked to confirm the results. The Vancouver group [8] developed ProMisE (Proactive Molecular Risk Classifier for Endometrial Cancer), based on the TCGA genomic subgroups. This proposed molecular classification system assessed DNA mismatch repair, POLE mutation, and p53 mutational status in 319 endometrial cancer samples. They utilized immunohistochemistry (IHC) for assessing DNA mismatch repair protein (MMR) expression; considering deficient or loss of expression as mismatch repair deficient (MMR-D). **Figure 3** shows an immunohistochemical view of an endometrial cancer with loss of expression of MLH1 DNA mismatch repair protein (MLH1 is shown and PMS2 loss also occurred but is not shown), while **Figure 4** shows normal expression for MSH6 protein (both MSH2 and MSH6 showed retained expression and only MSH6 is shown). They also assessed for POLE-mutation via DNA sequencing for polymerase-epsilon exonuclease domain mutation (POLE EDMs) and p53 mutation via IHC (wild-type expression or null/missense mutations,

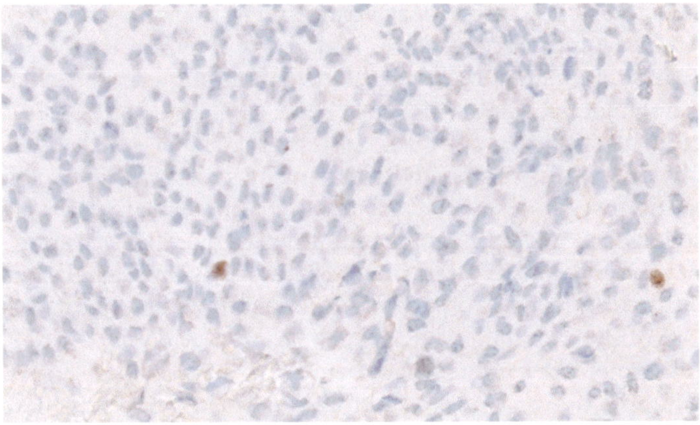

**Figure 3.**
*Loss of MLH1 immunoexpression.*

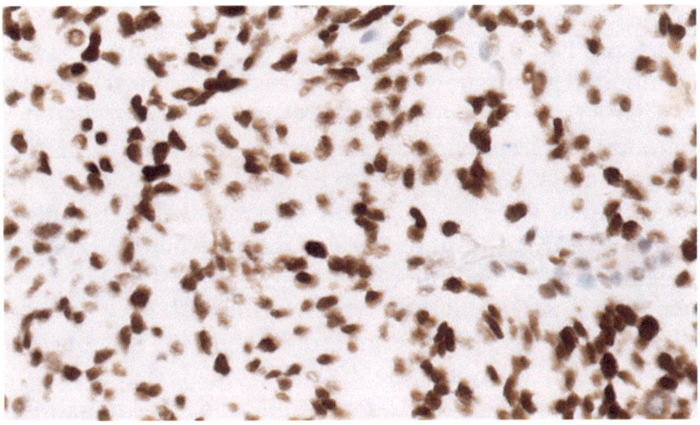

**Figure 4.**
*Retained MSH6 immunoexpression.*

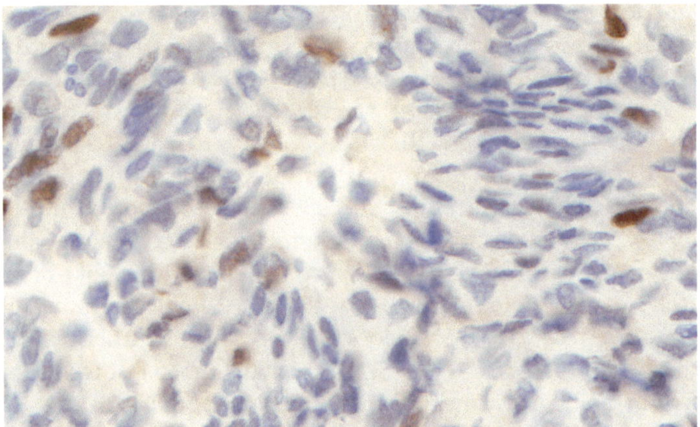

**Figure 5.**
*Normal (wild-type) p53 immunoexpression.*

termed p53 wt and p53 abn, respectively). **Figure 5** shows normal (termed wild-type) expression of the p53 protein in an endometrioid adenocarcinoma. **Figure 6** shows over-expression (mutant expression) in a serous carcinoma. **Figure 7** shows loss of expression (termed null phenotype) of p53 protein in another serous carcinoma. Authors in the Vancouver group were able to categorize all the endometrial cancer cases into the 4 prognostic subgroups; each with its own distinct disease-specific and progression-free survival, with statistical significance of $p < 0.001$. Overall, tumors with POLE EDMs had the most favorable prognosis, while the prognosis for tumors with pathogenic p53 mutations (p53 abn) was the worst. The other two molecular groups (DNA mismatch repair deficient group and the no specific molecular profile group) had comparatively intermediate prognosis. The authors next compared their ProMisE classifier system with the then-existing risk-stratification system of the European Society of Medical Oncology (ESMO). They found that while the ESMO system did not find survival differences between their low-risk and intermediate-risk

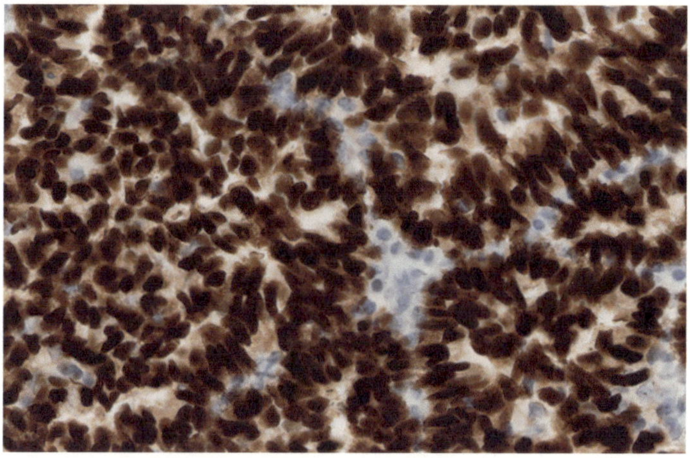

**Figure 6.**
*P53 over-expression (mutant) by immunohistochemistry.*

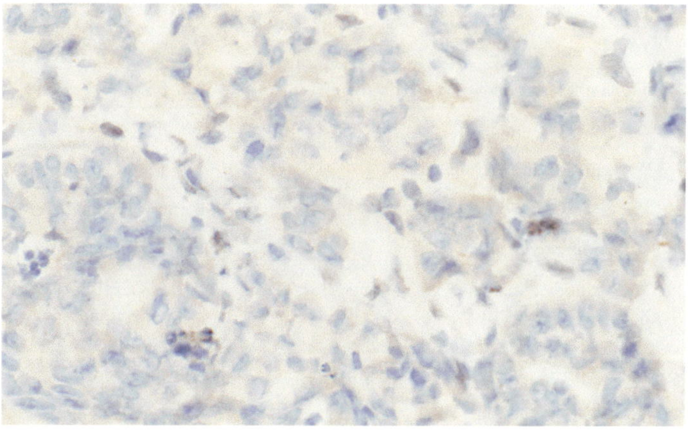

**Figure 7.**
*Loss of p53 immunoexpression (null phenotype).*

groups, the ProMisE system showed greater discriminating ability for outcomes. While there was overlap (89%) among the ProMisE p53 abn and the ESMO high-risk subgroups, there were otherwise no predictable associations between the molecular and ESMO risk groups. Thus the molecular classification system appeared to be not only prognostically different, but also showed differing therapeutic responses that were not evaluable using the then-existing classification.

## 4. Staging and prognostication of endometrial cancers

At the time of the new molecular proposal, the International Federation of Gynecology and Obstetrics (FIGO) 2009 staging system was in existence. Guidelines for endometrial cancer management were based on this staging scheme and are nicely summarized in the Colombo et al. paper [9]. Recurrence risk was based on histological subtype and tumor stage, and included the following data: high-grade (grade 3) histology, deep myometrial invasion (greater than or equal to 50% distinguishing stage 1A less than 50%, from stage 1B equal to or greater than 50%), presence of lymphovascular space invasion, lymph node metastases, and tumor size greater than 2 cm. **Table 1** summarizes the recurrence risk features used at that time. In addition, surgery and post-surgical management decisions were based on the FIGO 2009 staging system which incorporated data on tumor type and grade and stage as summarized

| Low risk | Low-grade histology (G1, G2), Endometrioid subtype, Low stage (1A) |
|---|---|
| Intermediate Risk | High-grade histology (G3), Endometrioid subtype, Low stage (1A) |
| High Risk | Low-grade histology (G1, G2), Endometrioid subtype, Higher stage (1B) |
| | High-grade histology (G3), Endometrioid subtype, Higher stage (1B) |
| | Non-endometrioid subtype, All stages |

**Table 1.**
*Recurrence risk categories for endometrial cancer in 2013.*

| FIGO 2009 | Histology | Surgical management |
|---|---|---|
| Stage I | 1A, G1–2 endometrioid carcinoma | TH/BSO |
| | 1A, G3 | TH/BSO +/− bilateral PPLND |
| | 1B, all grades (1,2,3) endometrioid | TH/BSO +/− bilateral PPLND |
| Stage II | All grades endometrioid | RH/BSO + bilateral PPLND |
| Stage III | All grades endometrioid | Maximal surgical cytoreduction |
| Stage IV | IVA endometrioid | Complete pelvic exenteration |
| | IVB endometrioid | Systemic therapy + palliative surgery |
| All stages | Non-endometrioid subtypes (serous, clear cell) | TH/BSO, PPLND, omentectomy, appendectomy, peritoneal biopsies<br>Platinum-based adjuvant chemotherapy |

*Abbreviations: TH/BSO – total hysterectomy, bilateral salpingooophorectomy, PPLND = pelvic and para-aortic lymphadenectomy, RH = radical hysterectomy.*

**Table 2.**
*Surgical management of endometrial cancer in 2013.*

| figo 2009 stage | Histology | Post surgical management |
|---|---|---|
| Stage I | IA, grades 1, 2<br>IA, grade 3 | Observation or vaginal BT<br>With (–) prognostic factors (age, LVSI, high tumor volume), pelvic RT +/– chemotherapy may be considered |
| | IB, grades 1,2 | Observation or vaginal BT<br>With (–) prognostic factors, pelvic RT +/– chemotherapy may be considered |
| | IB, grade 3 | Pelvic RT<br>With (–) prognostic factors, pelvic RT +/– chemotherapy may be considered |
| Stage II | | Pelvic RT and vaginal BT<br>If grade 1 or 2 tumor, myometrial invasions <50%, no LVSI and complete staging, BT only<br>If (–) prognostic factor, chemotherapy +/– radiation |
| Stage III, IV | | Chemotherapy<br>If positive LN, sequential radiotherapy<br>If metastatic disease, chemotherapy-RT for palliative management |

*Abbreviations: BT = brachytherapy, RT = radiation therapy, LVSI = lymphovascular space invasion, LN = lymph node.*

**Table 3.**
*Post-surgical management of endometrial cancer in 2013, using the FIGO 2009 staging criteria.*

| FIGO 2023 stage | Histologic type | Tumor features | Post surgical management |
|---|---|---|---|
| IA1 | Endometrioid, low-grade (G1, G2) | No myometrial invasion | Observation |
| IA2 | | <50% myoinvasion | Observation |
| IB | | > = 50% | Intravaginal radiation therapy (IVRT) |
| IC | High-grade endometrioid, serous, clear cell, MMT, dedifferentiated | No residual tumor | Observation |
| IC | | No myometrial invasion | IVRT, consider chemotherapy |
| IIC | | Myometrial invasion | IVRT, chemotherapy |
| IIC | | | |
| IIA | | | External beam radiation therapy (EBRT) |
| IIB | | LVSI >5 vessels | |
| IIIA1 | | Ovary, fallopian tube involvement | Chemotherapy* +/– RT<br>*Paclitaxel + Carboplatin + pembrolizumab, or paclitaxel, carboplatin + dostarlimab for MMRd<br>Her2 positive serous tumors consider adding trastuzumab to carboplatin and paclitaxel |
| IIIA2 | | Uterine serosa involved | |
| IIIB1 | | Vaginal involvement | Neoadjuvant chemotherapy, surgery, then EBRT after chemotherapy |
| IIIB1 | | Parametrial involvement | |
| IIIB2 | | Pelvic peritoneal involvement | |

| FIGO 2023 stage | Histologic type | Tumor features | Post surgical management |
|---|---|---|---|
| IIIC1 | Endometrioid, clear cell carcinomas | Pelvic lymph node involvement | Chemotherapy +/− IVRT<br>Consider immunotherapy, hormone therapy or other targeted therapy if appropriate |
| IIIC2 | | Para-aortic lymph node involvement | |
| IIIC1 | Serous, MMT, Dedifferentiated | Pelvic lymph nodes involved | Chemotherapy<br>Consider Immunotherapy, hormone therapy if tumor cells express appropriate targets |
| IIIC2 | | Para-aortic lymph nodes involved | |
| IVA | | Bladder / intestinal mucosal invasion | Chemotherapy +/− EBRT<br>Consider immunotherapy, hormone therapy or other targeted therapy if appropriate |
| IVB | | Abdominal / peritoneal metastases beyond pelvis | Primary cytoreduction vs. neoadjuvant chemotherapy Consider immunotherapy, hormone therapy or other targeted therapy if appropriate |
| IVC | | Distant metastasis (extra abdominal sites) +/− lymph nodes | Chemotherapy<br>Consider immunotherapy, hormone therapy or other targeted therapy if appropriate |

*LVSI = lymphovascular space invasion, MMT = mixed mullerian tumor, carcinosarcoma, RT = radiation therapy.*

**Table 4.**
*Post surgical management of endometrial cancers using the FIGO 2023 re-staging.*

in **Tables 2** and **3**. Staging of endometrial cancer by the International Federation of Gynecology and Obstetrics (FIGO) has undergone modifications with the advent of the new pathologic classification scheme, depicted in **Table 4** below, which also summarizes our thoughts on proposed management of the various stages, after discussion within our group. Note the enhanced stratification of tumor types enabled by the 4-tier pathologic classification system, and the greater precision in treating the different tumor types and stages, compared with the 2009 FIGO staging system.

The greater stratification of tumors within their stages using the 4-tier molecular classification system allows for: (i) improved reproducibility in pathologic diagnosis of high-grade endometrial cancers, (ii) improved stratification of patients for targeted therapy, clinical trials, (iii) better patient management, i.e., less over- and under-treatments administered, and (iv) identification of women at greater risk for having Lynch syndrome.

## 5. Targeted therapy

Around the time of the molecular classification proposal, immunotherapy was emerging as an FDA-approved method for the treatment of malignancy. This therapeutic modality has become a promising approach for patients who have targetable protein-expressing tumors. For example, for patients whose tumors exhibit DNA mismatch repair deficiency (MMR-D), Pembrolizumab is an immunoglobulin G4

(IgG4) kappa monoclonal antibody that binds to and inhibits T cell protein programmed death-1 (PD-1) receptor. PD-1 is found on the surface of T cells, natural killer cells and B cells. Tumor cells which express a programmed death ligand 1 (PD-L1) are able to bind to the PD-1 receptor on T cells and other immune surveillance cells. This interaction results in a negative regulatory signal which causes deactivation and downregulation of T cell effector activity; ultimately enabling PD-L1-expressing tumor cells to 'hide' from and avoid elimination by immune cells. By binding to and 'covering' the PD-1 receptors on T cells, pembrolizumab prevents the ability of PD-L1-expressing tumor cells to avoid immune surveillance, and thereby enables the normal T cell/immune cell pathway of elimination of tumor cells to occur [10, 11].

In cancers with a pathogenetic *TP53* gene mutation, the loss of tumor suppressor gene function allows for unchecked cell division and proliferation. Mutation of the *TP53* gene may be detected via p53 protein immunohistochemistry as was shown above in **Figures 5–7**. *TP53* gene-mutated endometrial cancers may also exhibit over-expression of the HER2/neu (c-erbB-2) protein. This protein is considered to be an oncogene and is a plasma membrane tyrosine kinase which, when activated plays an important role in cell proliferation, anti-apoptosis, and differentiation capabilities. When overexpressed, HER2 promotes rapid cancer cell growth and spread and as such, is another targetable protein in immune therapy. HER2 can be detected via HER2 immunostaining. **Figure 8** illustrates a HER2-expressing endometrial serous carcinoma. Note the strong, dark brown staining outlining the tumor cell plasma membranes. Criteria have been developed to guide pathologists in interpretation of the staining patterns to qualify a patient's tumor as clinically-relevant HER2-overexpressing. In doubtful cases, HER2 gene overexpression can be investigated by the use of fluorescence in situ hybridization (FISH).

Herceptin (trastuzumab) is a monoclonal antibody that specifically targets the HER2 receptor, binding to it and blocking the receptor's signaling pathway, which prevents further cell proliferation and marks the cancer cells for destruction by the immune system. It works by inhibiting AKT phosphorylation and arresting the cell cycle through AKT inhibition [12]. Additionally, patients in this group could be eligible for a newer, promising antibody-drug conjugate.

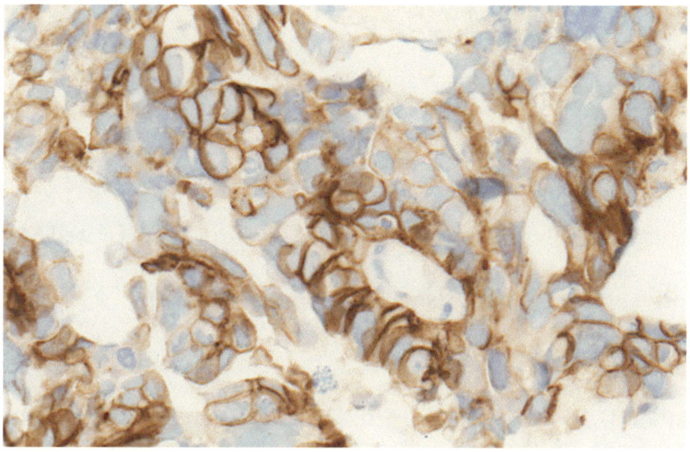

**Figure 8.**
*HER2 immunostained serous carcinoma.*

POLE mutated tumors generally have a positive prognosis due to their ultra mutated nature, which allows the immune system to detect them with greater ease [13]. Patients with POLE ultramutated tumors typically do not require aggressive therapeutic approaches such as chemotherapy or radiation. Instead, following up to monitor for any signs of recurrence or spread is felt to suffice. Patients with tumors without a specific mutational profile (NSMP) are more difficult to classify for precise treatment. These patients will typically follow the standard of care for treatments. While currently this cohort lacks the same targeted therapy recommendations, ongoing research will undoubtedly lend new insights into improved strategies.

## 6. Conclusion

In summary, the 4-tier molecular classification scheme for endometrial cancers has allowed for more accurate pathologic subtyping of these tumors, which in turn has enabled more detailed staging and management guidelines for endometrial cancer patients. We are a step closer to the ideal of precision medicine, wherein the treatment plan is tailored to the individual patient's tumor and unique clinical scenario.

## Thanks

A very special thanks to Alexandra Paul, who helped in the preparation of this manuscript.

## Author details

Tamara Kalir
The Icahn School of Medicine at Mount Sinai, New York City, United States

*Address all correspondence to: tamara.kalir@mountsinai.org

## References

[1] American Cancer Society. Available from: https://www.cancer.org/cancer/types/endometrial-cancer/about/key-statistics.html

[2] Bokhman JV. Two pathogenetic types of endometrial carcinoma. Gynecologic Oncology. 1983;**1983**(15):10-17

[3] Wang Y, Sun Y, Sun F, Han P, Fan R, Ren F. Comparison of clinical characteristics and prognosis between type I and type II endometrial cancer: A single-center retrospective study. Discover Oncology. 2023;**14**:211-223. DOI: 10.1007/s12672-023-00820-1

[4] Sherman ME, Bur ME, Kurman RJ. P53 in endometrial cancer and its putative precursors: Evidence for diverse pathways of tumorigenesis. Human Pathology. 1995;**26**:1268-1274. DOI: 10.1016/0046-8177(95)90204-x

[5] Lukanova A, Lundin E, Micheli A, Arsian A, Ferrari P, Rinaldi S, et al. Circulating levels of sex steroir hormones and risk of endometrial cancer in postmenopausal women. International Journal of Cancer. 2003;**108**:425-432. DOI: 10.1002/ijc.11529

[6] Gilks CB, Oliva E, Soslow RA. Poor interobserver reproducibility in the diagnosis of high-grade endometrial carcinoma. The American Journal of Surgical Pathology. 2013;**37**:874-881. DOI: 10.1097/PAS.0b013e31827f576a

[7] Levine DA, The Cancer Genome Atlas Research Network. Integrated genomic characterization of endometrial carcinoma. Nature. 2013;**2013**(497):67-73

[8] Talhouk A, McConechy MK, Leung S, Yang W, Lum A, Senz J, et al. Confirmation of ProMisE: A simple, genomics-based clinical classifier for endometrial cancer: Molecular classification of EC. Cancer. 2017;**123**: 802-813. DOI: 10.1002/cncr.30496

[9] Colombo N, Preti E, Landoni F, Carinelli S, Colombo A, Marini C, et al. Endometrial cancer: ESMO clinical practice guidelines for diagnosis, treatment and follow-up. Annals of Oncology. 2013;**24**(Suppl. 6):vi33-vi38. DOI: 10.1093/annonc/md353

[10] Dan TO, Ogunniyi A, Barbee MS, Drilon A. Pembrolizumab for the treatment of PD-L1 positive advanced or metastatic non-small cell lung cancer. Expert Review of Anticancer Therapy. 2016;**16**:13-20. DOI: 10.1586/14737140.2016.1123626

[11] Eskander RN, Sill MW, Beffa L, Moore RG, Hope JM, Musa FB, et al. Pembrolizumab plus chemotherapy in advanced endometrial cancer. New England Journal of Medicine [Internet]. 2023;**388**(23):2159-2170. Available from: https://www.nejm.org/doi/full/10.1056/NEJMoa2302312 [Accessed: September 14, 2024]

[12] Maadi H, Soheilifar MH, Choi WS, Moshtaghian A, Wang Z. Trastuzumab mechanism of action; 20 years of research to unravel a dilemma. Cancers (Basel) [Internet]. 2021;**13**(14):3540. Available from: https://www.ncbi.nlm.nih.gov/pmc/articles/PMC8303665/ [Accessed: September 14, 2024]

[13] Li Y, Bian Y, Wang K, Wan XP. POLE mutations improve the prognosis of endometrial cancer via regulating cellular metabolism through AMF/AMFR signal transduction. BMC Medical Genetics [Internet]. 2019;**20**(1):202. DOI: 10.1186/s12881-019-0936-2

## Chapter 4

# Staging in Cervical Cancer

*Merve Konal*


## Abstract

Cervical cancer remains a significant health concern globally, particularly in low- and middle-income countries. Accurate staging of cervical cancer is critical as it directly influences treatment decisions and prognostic assessments. This chapter provides a comprehensive overview of the staging methodologies used in cervical cancer, highlighting the International Federation of Gynecology and Obstetrics (FIGO) and the Tumor, Node, Metastasis (TNM) staging systems. It delves into diagnostic methods, including clinical examination, advanced imaging techniques, and pathological evaluation, and discusses recent advancements such as molecular imaging, biomarkers, and artificial intelligence. The chapter also explores the clinical implications of staging, including its role in treatment planning, prognostic evaluation, and follow-up care. Additionally, it addresses the challenges and future directions in cervical cancer staging, emphasizing the importance of emerging technologies and personalized medicine approaches. By enhancing the accuracy of staging, these advancements aim to improve patient outcomes and quality of life for those affected by cervical cancer.


**Keywords:** cervical cancer, staging, FIGO, TNM, imaging techniques, biopsy, biomarkers, artificial intelligence, personalized medicine, global health

## 1. Introduction

Cervical cancer remains one of the most common malignancies affecting women worldwide, particularly in low- and middle-income countries [1]. Accurate staging of cervical cancer is crucial as it directly influences treatment decisions and prognostic assessments [2]. The staging process involves a thorough evaluation of the tumor's size, depth of invasion, and spread to adjacent tissues or distant organs. This introductory section aims to provide a comprehensive overview of the staging methodologies used in cervical cancer, underscoring the importance of each stage in guiding clinical management [3].

The staging of cervical cancer has evolved significantly over the years, with advances in imaging techniques and pathological assessments enhancing the precision of diagnosis [4]. The most widely adopted system for staging cervical cancer is the International Federation of Gynecology and Obstetrics (FIGO) staging system, which has undergone several revisions to incorporate new clinical insights and technological advancements [5]. Understanding the nuances of this staging system is essential for both clinicians and researchers involved in the field of gynecologic oncology.

Historically, cervical cancer staging was primarily based on clinical examination findings, which often led to inaccuracies due to limitations in detecting the extent of the disease. However, with the advent of modern imaging techniques such as magnetic resonance imaging (MRI), computed tomography (CT), and positron emission tomography (PET), the ability to accurately stage cervical cancer has improved markedly [6, 7]. These imaging modalities allow for a more detailed assessment of tumor size, lymph node involvement, and distant metastases, thereby facilitating more precise staging and better-informed treatment decisions [8].

Another critical aspect of cervical cancer staging is the pathological evaluation of biopsy samples. Pathological staging provides definitive information about the tumor's histological type, grade, and the presence of lymphovascular space invasion, which are all crucial for accurate staging and treatment planning [9]. Biopsy samples from the cervix, as well as from suspicious lymph nodes, help determine the extent of disease spread and inform decisions regarding surgical or radiotherapeutic interventions [10].

In addition to traditional clinical and pathological staging methods, recent advances in molecular biology have introduced new biomarkers that may improve the precision of cervical cancer staging. Biomarkers such as HPV DNA, p16INK4a, and Ki-67 have shown promise in providing additional prognostic information and may eventually be integrated into standard staging protocols [11]. These molecular markers can help identify high-risk patients who may benefit from more aggressive treatment strategies, thereby potentially improving outcomes.

The introduction of artificial intelligence (AI) and machine learning techniques in imaging and pathology is also revolutionizing cervical cancer staging. AI algorithms can analyze imaging data and histopathological slides with high accuracy, potentially identifying subtle features that may be overlooked by human observers [12]. These technologies have the potential to enhance staging accuracy and consistency, ultimately leading to more personalized and effective treatment plans [13].

Despite these advancements, several challenges remain in the staging of cervical cancer. Discrepancies between clinical and pathological staging, variations in imaging interpretation, and the need for standardized protocols across different healthcare settings can complicate the staging process. Moreover, access to advanced imaging and molecular diagnostic tools may be limited in resource-poor settings, highlighting the need for globally applicable and cost-effective staging methods [14].

In conclusion, accurate staging of cervical cancer is fundamental to effective clinical management and improved patient outcomes. The ongoing evolution of staging methodologies, driven by technological advancements and molecular insights, holds great promise for the future of cervical cancer care. This chapter will delve into the various staging systems, diagnostic methods, and emerging technologies that are shaping the field of cervical cancer staging, providing a comprehensive guide for clinicians and researchers alike.

## 2. Staging systems for cervical cancer

### 2.1 International federation of gynecology and obstetrics (FIGO) staging system

The FIGO staging system is the most widely used classification for cervical cancer staging. It provides a standardized approach to evaluate the extent of disease, helping to guide treatment decisions and predict patient outcomes [2]. The FIGO system categorizes cervical cancer into stages I through IV, with further subdivisions to reflect the progressive severity and spread of the disease (**Table 1**) [3].

*DOI: http://dx.doi.org/10.5772/intechopen.1006545*

| Parameter | GnRH agonists | GnRH antagonists |
|---|---|---|
| Initial hormone surge | Present | Absent |
| Time to suppression | Delayed | Immediate |
| Menopausal symptoms | Common | Less common |
| Bone density loss | Significant | Moderate |
| Efficacy in pain reduction | High | High |

**Table 1.**
*Comparison of side effects and efficacy between GnRH agonists and antagonists.*

Stage I represents cancer confined to the cervix, whereas Stage II indicates extension beyond the cervix but not to the pelvic wall or lower third of the vagina. Stage III involves spread to the pelvic wall and/or the lower third of the vagina, and Stage IV indicates invasion into the bladder or rectum, or distant metastasis [4]. Each stage is further divided into subcategories (e.g., IA, IB, and IIA) based on specific criteria such as tumor size and involvement of specific tissues [5].

Historically, FIGO staging relied heavily on clinical examination, which included inspection, palpation, colposcopy, endocervical curettage, and radiographic examinations [6]. However, advancements in imaging techniques have been incorporated into the staging process, improving the accuracy of the FIGO system [7]. For instance, MRI is now frequently used to assess tumor size and local extension, while CT and PET scans help evaluate lymph node involvement and distant metastases [10].

## 2.2 TNM staging system

The Tumor, Node, Metastasis (TNM) staging system, developed by the American Joint Committee on Cancer (AJCC), is another widely used classification method (**Table 2**). This system considers the size and local extent of the primary tumor (T), the involvement of regional lymph nodes (N), and the presence of distant metastasis (M) [2]. The TNM system provides a detailed framework for assessing the anatomical spread of cervical cancer and is often used in conjunction with the FIGO system to provide a more comprehensive assessment of the disease [7].

In the TNM system, the primary tumor (T) is classified from T1 to T4, based on its size and extent of local invasion. Regional lymph nodes (N) are categorized from N0 (no regional lymph node involvement) to N3 (extensive regional lymph node involvement). Distant metastasis (M) is classified as either M0 (no distant metastasis) or M1 (presence of distant metastasis) [15].

| Drug | Efficacy in pain reduction (%) | Reduction in lesion size (%) | Common side effects |
|---|---|---|---|
| Medroxyprogesterone acetate | 70 | 60 | Weight gain, mood changes |
| Norethindrone acetate | 75 | 65 | Breakthrough bleeding |
| Dienogest | 80 | 70 | Headache, breast tenderness |
| Ulipristal acetate | 85 | 75 | Nausea, abdominal pain |

**Table 2.**
*Clinical outcomes of different progestins and SPRMs in the treatment of endometriosis.*

One of the advantages of the TNM system is its ability to incorporate findings from modern imaging techniques and pathological examinations, providing a more nuanced understanding of disease spread [15]. For instance, sentinel lymph node biopsy and advanced imaging modalities such as PET/CT scans can provide detailed information about lymph node involvement and distant metastases, enhancing the accuracy of TNM staging [10].

Both the FIGO and TNM staging systems are essential tools in the clinical management of cervical cancer. They provide a common language for healthcare professionals to describe the extent of disease, guide treatment decisions, and predict patient outcomes. Understanding the strengths and limitations of each system is crucial for optimizing patient care and improving prognostic assessments [16].

## 3. Diagnostic methods for staging

### 3.1 Clinical examination

Clinical examination remains a fundamental component of cervical cancer staging. It involves a thorough pelvic examination to assess the size and spread of the tumor, as well as the potential involvement of adjacent structures [3]. The examination typically includes inspection, palpation, and the use of a speculum to visualize the cervix. Despite its limitations in detecting microscopic disease and accurately assessing tumor size, clinical examination is essential for initial staging and guiding further diagnostic procedures [17].

### 3.2 Imaging techniques

Advancements in imaging techniques have significantly improved the accuracy of cervical cancer staging. Various imaging modalities provide detailed information about the tumor and its spread, enhancing the precision of staging.

#### *3.2.1 Magnetic resonance imaging (MRI)*

MRI is particularly valuable for assessing tumor size and local invasion. It provides high-resolution images of soft tissues, allowing for detailed evaluation of the cervical tumor and its relationship to surrounding structures. MRI is considered the imaging modality of choice for local staging of cervical cancer due to its superior contrast resolution compared to other techniques. MRI can also detect parametrical invasion and involvement of adjacent organs, which are critical factors in staging and treatment planning [8].

#### *3.2.2 Computed tomography (CT) scans*

CT scans are used to detect lymph node involvement and distant metastases. They provide cross-sectional images of the body, which can help identify enlarged lymph nodes and potential sites of metastatic spread [7]. Although CT is less effective than MRI in assessing local tumor extent, it is useful for evaluating distant disease. CT scans are often used in combination with other imaging modalities to provide a comprehensive assessment of disease spread [10].

#### *3.2.3 Positron emission tomography (PET) scans*

PET scans provide functional imaging to identify the metabolic activity of cancer cells. By detecting areas of increased glucose metabolism, PET can reveal both primary and metastatic tumor sites that may not be visible on other imaging modalities [11]. PET/CT, a combination of PET and CT, is often used for comprehensive staging and restaging of cervical cancer. This combined approach improves the accuracy of detecting lymph node involvement and distant metastases, providing valuable information for treatment planning [10].

#### *3.2.4 Ultrasonography*

Ultrasonography is a non-invasive imaging technique that can be used to evaluate the pelvic organs. Transvaginal ultrasonography is particularly useful for initial assessment of cervical tumors and for guiding biopsies [8]. Although less detailed than MRI or CT, ultrasonography is a valuable tool in resource-limited settings due to its accessibility and cost-effectiveness [14].

### 3.3 Pathological evaluation

#### *3.3.1 Biopsy*

Biopsy is the gold standard for diagnosing cervical cancer and provides crucial information for staging. Tissue samples obtained through biopsy are examined histologically to determine the type and grade of the tumor [18]. Pathological evaluation also helps identify the presence of lymphovascular space invasion, which is an important prognostic factor [15]. Different biopsy techniques, such as punch biopsy, cone biopsy, and endocervical curettage, may be used depending on the clinical scenario [16].

#### *3.3.2 Lymph node assessment*

Assessment of lymph node involvement is critical for accurate staging and treatment planning. Sentinel lymph node biopsy and pelvic lymphadenectomy are common procedures used to evaluate regional lymph nodes [17]. The presence of cancer cells in the lymph nodes often indicates a more advanced stage and may necessitate additional treatments such as chemotherapy or radiotherapy [19]. Recent advances in imaging techniques, such as PET/CT, have enhanced the ability to detect lymph node metastases non-invasively, improving the accuracy of staging [10].

These diagnostic methods collectively contribute to a more accurate and comprehensive staging of cervical cancer. The integration of clinical examination, advanced imaging techniques, and pathological evaluation provides a robust framework for staging, guiding treatment decisions, and improving patient outcomes [20].

## 4. Advances in staging techniques

### 4.1 Molecular imaging

Molecular imaging techniques, such as PET with novel tracers, are being explored to improve the sensitivity and specificity of cervical cancer staging. These advanced

| Pain management strategy | Type | Effectiveness in pain reduction (%) | Common side effects |
|---|---|---|---|
| NSAIDs | Pharmacological | 70 | GI issues |
| Opioids | Pharmacological | 80 | Dependency |
| Neuromodulators | Pharmacological | 75 | Drowsiness |
| Acupuncture | Non-pharmacological | 60 | None |
| Physical therapy | Non-pharmacological | 65 | Muscle soreness |

**Table 3.**
*Overview of pharmacological and non-pharmacological pain management strategies.*

imaging methods can detect molecular and cellular changes associated with cancer, providing earlier and more accurate staging information [21]. Molecular imaging has the potential to identify occult metastases and guide targeted therapies, enhancing personalized treatment approaches [22].

### 4.2 Biomarkers in staging

Biomarkers, including HPV DNA, p16INK4a, and Ki-67, have shown potential in enhancing the staging of cervical cancer (**Table 3**). These biomarkers can provide additional prognostic information and help identify high-risk patients who may benefit from more aggressive treatment strategies. Integration of biomarker analysis into routine clinical practice may improve the accuracy of staging and tailor treatment to individual patient profiles [23].

### 4.3 Artificial intelligence in imaging

Artificial intelligence (AI) and machine learning are increasingly being applied to medical imaging for cervical cancer staging. AI algorithms can analyze imaging data and histopathological slides with high accuracy, potentially identifying subtle features that may be overlooked by human observers. These technologies have the potential to enhance staging accuracy and consistency, leading to more personalized and effective treatment plans.

AI can also assist in the standardization of imaging interpretation, reducing inter-observer variability and ensuring consistent application of staging criteria across different healthcare settings. The integration of AI into clinical workflows represents a significant advancement in the field of cervical cancer staging and has the potential to improve patient outcomes.

These advances in staging techniques are reshaping the landscape of cervical cancer diagnosis and management. By incorporating molecular imaging, biomarkers, and artificial intelligence, clinicians can achieve more accurate staging, leading to better-informed treatment decisions and improved prognostic assessments [24].

## 5. Clinical implications of staging

### 5.1 Treatment planning

Accurate staging is essential for effective treatment planning in cervical cancer. The stage of the disease determines the choice of treatment modalities, which may

| Stage | Treatment modality |
|---|---|
| Stage I | Surgery (e.g., radical hysterectomy) |
| Stage II | Combination of surgery and radiotherapy or chemoradiotherapy |
| Stage III | Chemoradiotherapy |
| Stage IV | Palliative care, chemotherapy, targeted therapy |

**Table 4.**
*Treatment modalities based on cervical cancer staging.*

include surgery, radiotherapy, chemotherapy, or a combination of these approaches. For instance, early-stage cervical cancer (Stage I) is often treated with surgery alone, such as a radical hysterectomy. In contrast, locally advanced stages (Stages II-III) may require a combination of radiotherapy and chemotherapy to control the disease. In advanced stages (Stage IV), palliative treatments are often employed to alleviate symptoms and improve quality of life (**Table 4**).

The integration of accurate staging information allows oncologists to tailor treatment plans to the individual patient, maximizing therapeutic efficacy while minimizing unnecessary side effects. For example, the identification of lymph node metastasis through advanced imaging techniques can prompt the use of adjuvant chemoradiotherapy, which has been shown to improve survival outcomes [15].

### 5.2 Prognostic value

Staging provides critical prognostic information, helping to predict patient outcomes and guide follow-up care. Higher stages of cervical cancer are associated with poorer prognosis and increased risk of recurrence, emphasizing the importance of accurate staging in clinical practice. For example, patients with Stage I disease have a significantly higher 5-year survival rate compared to those with Stage IV disease.

Prognostic factors such as tumor size, lymph node involvement, and depth of invasion are integral components of staging systems and provide valuable insights into disease progression. Accurate staging enables clinicians to stratify patients based on their risk profiles and implement appropriate surveillance strategies [25].

### 5.3 Follow-up and surveillance

Accurate staging also informs follow-up and surveillance strategies. Patients with early-stage disease may require less intensive follow-up compared to those with advanced-stage disease, who may need more frequent monitoring for recurrence and metastasis. Follow-up protocols typically include regular clinical examinations, imaging studies, and cytological assessments to detect any signs of disease recurrence.

For patients with advanced-stage disease or those who have received multimodal treatments, follow-up care may involve more frequent visits and comprehensive evaluations, including PET/CT scans and biomarker analyses. These measures help in early detection of recurrence, allowing for timely intervention and improved management of the disease.

The clinical implications of staging extend beyond initial treatment and include long-term management and survivorship care. By understanding the stage-specific risks and potential complications, healthcare providers can deliver personalized follow-up care, ultimately enhancing patient outcomes and quality of life [26].

## 6. Challenges and future directions

### 6.1 Limitations of current staging systems

Despite advancements in staging techniques, current staging systems have several limitations. One major challenge is the discrepancy between clinical and pathological staging, which can lead to inconsistencies in treatment planning. Clinical staging, which relies heavily on physical examination and basic imaging, may underestimate the extent of disease compared to pathological staging, which includes detailed histological evaluation.

Variations in imaging interpretation also pose challenges, as different radiologists may provide different assessments of tumor size and spread based on the same set of images. This inter-observer variability can affect the accuracy of staging and, consequently, the treatment approach. Additionally, the lack of standardized protocols across different healthcare settings can lead to variability in staging practices and outcomes [27].

### 6.2 Emerging technologies

Emerging technologies hold promise for overcoming some of the limitations of current staging systems. Next-generation sequencing (NGS) and liquid biopsy techniques are being explored to provide more detailed genetic and molecular profiles of tumors. These advanced diagnostic tools can detect circulating tumor DNA (ctDNA) and other biomarkers in the blood, offering non-invasive methods for staging and monitoring disease progression.

Liquid biopsy, in particular, has the potential to detect microscopic metastases and minimal residual disease that are not visible on conventional imaging. This technology could revolutionize cervical cancer staging by providing real-time insights into tumor dynamics and treatment response, enabling more precise and personalized therapeutic strategies [28].

### 6.3 Personalized medicine approaches

The future of cervical cancer staging lies in personalized medicine approaches, where staging and treatment are tailored to the individual patient based on genetic, molecular, and clinical factors. Personalized medicine aims to move beyond the traditional one-size-fits-all approach and considers the unique characteristics of each patient's cancer.

For example, molecular subtyping of cervical cancer based on gene expression profiles can identify distinct subgroups with different prognoses and treatment responses. This information can guide the selection of targeted therapies and immunotherapies, improving treatment efficacy and reducing unnecessary toxicity.

Artificial intelligence and machine learning algorithms can also play a crucial role in personalized medicine by analyzing large datasets and identifying patterns that are not apparent to human observers. These technologies can integrate genomic, imaging, and clinical data to develop predictive models for treatment response and disease progression, supporting more informed clinical decision-making [29].

### 6.4 Global Health considerations

Addressing global health disparities is a critical challenge in cervical cancer staging. Access to advanced imaging and molecular diagnostic tools is often limited in low- and middle-income countries, where the burden of cervical cancer is the highest. Efforts to improve global health equity should focus on increasing access to essential diagnostic and staging tools, as well as implementing cost-effective and scalable solutions.

Training and capacity-building initiatives are also essential to ensure that healthcare providers in resource-limited settings can effectively utilize available technologies and adhere to standardized staging protocols. International collaborations and partnerships can facilitate the sharing of knowledge, resources, and best practices, ultimately improving cervical cancer care worldwide.

In conclusion, while significant progress has been made in cervical cancer staging, ongoing challenges and emerging opportunities highlight the need for continued innovation and collaboration. By embracing new technologies and personalized medicine approaches, and addressing global health disparities, we can improve the accuracy of staging and outcomes for patients with cervical cancer [30].

## 7. Conclusion

Accurate staging of cervical cancer is a cornerstone of effective clinical management, guiding treatment decisions and providing critical prognostic information. Over the years, the staging of cervical cancer has evolved significantly, with advancements in imaging techniques, pathological assessments, and molecular diagnostics enhancing the precision of staging.

The International Federation of Gynecology and Obstetrics (FIGO) and the Tumor, Node, Metastasis (TNM) staging systems remain the primary frameworks for classifying the extent of cervical cancer. These systems, complemented by clinical examination and advanced imaging modalities such as MRI, CT, and PET scans, provide a comprehensive assessment of the disease. Pathological evaluation, including biopsy and lymph node assessment, further refines the staging process, offering crucial insights into tumor characteristics and spread.

Emerging technologies, such as molecular imaging, biomarkers, and artificial intelligence, are poised to revolutionize cervical cancer staging. These innovations promise to improve staging accuracy, personalize treatment strategies, and ultimately enhance patient outcomes. Molecular imaging techniques and biomarkers offer new avenues for detecting occult metastases and tailoring therapies to individual patient profiles, while AI and machine learning algorithms provide powerful tools for integrating and analyzing complex datasets.

Despite these advancements, challenges remain. Discrepancies between clinical and pathological staging, variability in imaging interpretation, and the need for standardized protocols across different healthcare settings can complicate the staging process. Addressing these challenges requires continued innovation, collaboration, and efforts to improve global health equity. Ensuring that healthcare providers in resource-limited settings have access to essential diagnostic tools and training is crucial for advancing cervical cancer care worldwide.

In conclusion, the ongoing evolution of cervical cancer staging methodologies, driven by technological advancements and molecular insights, holds great promise for the future. By embracing new technologies, personalized medicine approaches, and addressing global health disparities, we can improve the accuracy of staging and outcomes for patients with cervical cancer. This comprehensive approach will enable clinicians and researchers to better understand the disease, develop more effective treatments, and ultimately improve the quality of life for patients affected by cervical cancer.

## Acknowledgements

The author acknowledges the use of ChatGPT for language polishing of the manuscript.

## Conflict of interest

The authors declare no conflict of interest.

## Author details

Merve Konal
Hitit University Erol Olçok Training and Research Hospital, Department of Obstetrics and Gynecology, Gynecologic Oncology Department, Çorum, Turkey

*Address all correspondence to: mervekonal@gmail.com

**IntechOpen**

## References

[1] Bhatla N, Aoki D, Sharma DN, Sankaranarayanan R. Cancer of the cervix uteri. International Journal of Gynaecology and Obstetrics. 2018;**143**:22-36

[2] Cibula D, Pötter R, Planchamp F, et al. The European Society of Gynaecological Oncology/European Society for Radiotherapy and Oncology/European Society of Pathology Guidelines for the Management of Patients with Cervical Cancer. International Journal of Gynecological Cancer. 2018;**28**:641-655

[3] Cohen PA, Jhingran A, Oaknin A, Denny L. Cervical cancer. Lancet. 2019;**393**:169-182

[4] Gadducci A, Guerrieri ME. Immune checkpoint inhibitors in Gynecological cancers: Update of literature and perspectives of clinical research. Anticancer Research. 2017;**37**:5955-5965

[5] Long X, He M, Yang L, et al. Validation of the 2018 FIGO staging system for predicting the prognosis of patients with stage IIIC cervical cancer. Clinical Medicine Insights: Oncology. 2023;**17**:11795549221146652

[6] Kessler TA. Cervical cancer: Prevention and early detection. Seminars in Oncology Nursing. 2017;**33**:172-183

[7] Koh WJ, Abu-Rustum NR, Bean S, et al. Cervical cancer, version 3.2019, NCCN clinical practice guidelines in oncology. Journal of the National Comprehensive Cancer Network. 2019;**17**:64-84

[8] Kim YB, Ghosh K, Ainbinder S, Berek JS. Diagnostic and therapeutic advances in gynecologic oncology: Screening for gynecologic cancer. Cancer Treatment and Research. 1998;**95**:253-276

[9] Gil-Ibañez B, Gil-Moreno A, Torné A, et al. Tumor size and oncological outcomes in patients with early cervical cancer treated by fertility preservation surgery: A Multicenter retrospective cohort study. Cancers (Basel). 2022;**14**:2108

[10] Nguyen NC, Beriwal S, Moon CH, et al. Diagnostic value of FDG PET/MRI in females with pelvic malignancy-a systematic review of the literature. Frontiers in Oncology. 2020;**10**:519440

[11] Meijer CJ, Berkhof J, Castle PE, et al. Guidelines for human papillomavirus DNA test requirements for primary cervical cancer screening in women 30 years and older. International Journal of Cancer. 2009;**124**:516-520

[12] Monk BJ, Tewari KS, Koh WJ. Multimodality therapy for locally advanced cervical carcinoma: State of the art and future directions. Journal of Clinical Oncology. 2007;**25**:2952-2965

[13] Poddar P, Maheshwari A. Surgery for cervical cancer: Consensus and controversies. The Indian Journal of Medical Research. 2021;**154**:284-292

[14] Bosse T, Lax S, Abu-Rustum N, Matias-Guiu X. The role of predictive biomarkers in Endocervical adenocarcinoma: Recommendations from the International Society of Gynecological Pathologists. International Journal of Gynecological Pathology. 2021;**40**:102-110

[15] Olawaiye AB, Baker TP, Washington MK, Mutch DG. The new (version 9) American joint committee on

cancer tumor, node, metastasis staging for cervical cancer. CA: a Cancer Journal for Clinicians. 2021;**71**:287-298

[16] Knoth J, Pötter R, Jürgenliemk-Schulz IM, et al. Clinical and imaging findings in cervical cancer and their impact on FIGO and TNM staging - an analysis from the EMBRACE study. Gynecologic Oncology. 2020;**159**:136-141

[17] Petignat P, Roy M. Diagnosis and management of cervical cancer. BMJ. 2007;**335**:765-768

[18] Okunade KS. Human papillomavirus and cervical cancer. Journal of Obstetrics and Gynaecology. 2020;**40**(5):602-608

[19] Pötter R, Tanderup K, Schmid MP, et al. MRI-guided adaptive brachytherapy in locally advanced cervical cancer (EMBRACE-I): A multicentre prospective cohort study. The Lancet Oncology. 2021;**22**:538-547

[20] Quinn MA, Benedet JL, Odicino F, et al. Carcinoma of the cervix uteri. FIGO 26th annual report on the results of treatment in Gynecological cancer. International Journal of Gynaecology and Obstetrics. 2006;**95**:43-103

[21] Salani R, Khanna N, Frimer M, Bristow RE, Chen LM. An update on post-treatment surveillance and diagnosis of recurrence in women with gynecologic malignancies: Society of Gynecologic Oncology (SGO) recommendations. Gynecologic Oncology. 2017;**146**:3-10

[22] Wright JD, Matsuo K, Huang Y, et al. Prognostic performance of the 2018 international federation of gynecology and obstetrics cervical cancer staging guidelines. Obstetrics and Gynecology. 2019;**134**:49-57

[23] Li Y, Liu J, Gong L, Sun X, Long W. Combining HPV DNA load with p16/Ki-67 staining to detect cervical precancerous lesions and predict the progression of CIN1-2 lesions. Virology Journal. 2019;**16**:117

[24] Bedell SL, Goldstein LS, Goldstein AR, Goldstein AT. Cervical cancer screening: Past, present, and future. Sexual Medicine Reviews. 2020;**8**:28-37

[25] Weyl A, Illac C, Lusque A, et al. Prognostic value of lymphovascular space invasion in early-stage cervical cancer. International Journal of Gynecological Cancer. 2020;**30**:1493-1499

[26] Lycke KD, Kahlert J, Petersen LK, et al. Untreated cervical intraepithelial neoplasia grade 2 and subsequent risk of cervical cancer: Population based cohort study. BMJ. 2023;**383**:e075925

[27] Mayadev JS, Ke G, Mahantshetty U, Pereira MD, Tarnawski R, Toita T. Global challenges of radiotherapy for the treatment of locally advanced cervical cancer. International Journal of Gynecological Cancer. 2022;**32**:436-445

[28] Hamashima C. Emerging technologies for cervical cancer screening. Japanese Journal of Clinical Oncology. 2021;**51**:1462-1470

[29] Willows K, Selk A, Auclair MH, et al. 2023 Canadian colposcopy guideline: A risk-based approach to management and surveillance of cervical dysplasia. Current Oncology. 2023;**30**:5738-5768

[30] Sung H, Ferlay J, Siegel RL, et al. Global cancer statistics 2020: GLOBOCAN estimates of incidence and mortality worldwide for 36 cancers in 185 countries. CA: A Cancer Journal for Clinicians. 2021;**71**:209-249

Chapter 5

# Do Vegetarian Dietary Patterns Affect the Risk of Breast Cancer?

*Pegah Hadi Sichani, Maede Makhtoomi, Masoud Amini Kahrizsangi, Zainab Shateri, Mehran Nouri and Marzieh Mahmoodi*

## Abstract

Breast cancer is the second most common cancer and one of the most common cancers in women worldwide. Breast cancer is known as a multifactorial disease in which several factors play a role in its occurrence. The risk factors of this cancer can be classified into two categories, non-modifiable and modifiable. It has been shown that modifiable lifestyle factors, such as diet, play an important role in cancer prevention. Recently, instead of using specific foods as indicators of dietary intake and nutritional status, component food group analysis has been used to determine dietary patterns. Although the findings are insufficient to evaluate the relationship between diet and breast cancer risk, a reduction in breast cancer risk has been reported following an increase in fruit and vegetable consumption. Adherence to vegetarian dietary patterns is associated with an increase in the consumption of plant-based foods and a decrease in the consumption of red meat and processed meat. It seems that vegetarian diets may have a potential role in alleviating the development and progression of breast cancer through their several anticancer properties. However, more studies are suggested to investigate the clear and comprehensive mechanism by comparing the effect of a vegetarian diet and a nonvegetarian diet on breast cancer risk in premenopausal and postmenopausal women.

**Keywords:** vegetarian dietary patterns, vegetarian diet, food patterns, breast cancer, breast neoplasms

## 1. Introduction

Breast cancer is known as the abnormal growth of breast cells, which means that the development of these cells goes out of control and turns into a tumor. This tumor can be benign and is often not life-threatening, or it can be malignant, which causes these cells to spread to breast tissue, lymph nodes, and other organs, leading to an increased risk of fatality through metastasis [1].

Common classifications used for invasive breast cancer include estrogen receptor (ER), progesterone receptor (PR), and human epidermal growth factor receptor 2 (HER2). These classifications are based on various factors such as etiology, clinical presentation, molecular characteristics, and response to treatment [2].

Although the recent attention on molecular classifications of breast cancer has been due to the very elegant, prognostic, and predictive nature of molecular and genetic tests, it is extensive and not yet widely available. Additionally, despite the diagnostic information obtained from molecular testing, reports of assay results provide little specific guidance on the response to targeted and proven therapy. However, the immunohistochemistry (IHC) classification and therapeutic and prognostic information are inexpensive and readily available [3].

## 2. Prevalence of breast cancer

Breast cancer is the second most common cancer [2] and one of the most common cancers in women worldwide, and its incidence is increasing in all regions of the world. However, the highest incidence is reported in industrialized countries [4]. As much as half of the cases are in developed countries [4]. This increase in incidence is attributed to the Western lifestyle, which is related to poor diet, excessive stress, and little physical activity [4].

In 2012, approximately 1.67 million people were reported to have been diagnosed with breast cancer, accounting for 25% of all cancers [2]. Approximately 2.089 million women with breast cancer were reported in 2018 [4]. The incidence rate of breast cancer ranges from 27 per 100,000 in Middle Africa and East Asia to 92 per 100,000 in North America [2].

An estimated incidence rate of 3.2 million people by 2050 has also been proposed [2, 5]. Since the population of elderly people is increasing in developed countries, it has been shown that the incidence rate of cancer in elderly people is increasing [2, 5]. According to reports in 2017, there were approximately 252,710 new cases of invasive breast cancer and 6341 cases of breast cancer in situ in the United States [2]. About 24% of breast cancer cases are reported in the Asia Pacific region with the highest incidence in Japan, China, and Indonesia [2, 6, 7]. The incidence rate of breast cancer (age-standardized rate per 100,000) in different regions of the world, such as more developed regions, less developed regions, Western Europe, Northern America, Northern Europe, Australia/New Zealand, South-Central Asia, and Eastern Asia, was reported to be 74.1, 31.3, 96, 91.6, 89.4, 85.8, 28.2, and 27, respectively [2].

According to evidence, 16,967 new cases of breast cancer and 4810 deaths related to breast cancer were reported in Iran in 2020 [8, 9]. Iran's cancer registry data from 2008 to 2016 has reported that the incidence of breast cancer in women will increase by 63% by 2025 [8, 10].

## 3. Breast cancer risk factors

Breast cancer is known as a multifactorial disease in which several factors play a role in its occurrence [2]. Population structure, lifestyle, genetic factors, and the environment are all known influencing factors [2, 5]. Variations in disease risk factors increase its prevalence, which is growing daily [2]. In general, disease risk factors are divided into inherent and extrinsic categories [11]. Age, race, and genetics are considered intrinsic risk factors, while lifestyle and diet are extrinsic risk factors [11]. In another classification, risk factors are classified into non-modifiable and modifiable categories [12]. In this way, older age (more than 65 versus less than 65 years old), genetic predisposition including deoxyribonucleic acid (DNA) mutation and breast cancer family history, early menarche (less than 12 years old), late menopause (more than 55 years old), age at first pregnancy over 30 years, infertility and childlessness, use of contraceptives, hormonal treatment after menopause, and no history of breastfeeding are included in the category of non-modifiable risk factors [12, 13]. Lifestyle, including food choices and being obese or overweight, is also included in the category of modifiable risk factors [12, 14, 15].

## 4. Nutritional aspects of breast cancer

It has been shown that modifiable lifestyle factors, such as diet, play an important role in cancer prevention [16]. As mentioned, diet is known as a modifiable factor among cancer risk factors [17]. Findings obtained from assessing the relationship between various single foods and nutrients and breast cancer have reported that dietary changes prevent about one-third of breast cancer cases [17]. Therefore, adherence to a healthier diet pattern that is nutrient-dense and has fewer energy-dense foods has been emphasized [17, 18]. In this view, the relationship between the consumption of a poor nutrient diet and energy-dense foods with the risk of breast cancer has been shown [16, 19].

The World Cancer Research Fund (WCRF) also emphasizes adherence to this healthy eating pattern, which has been suggested as a way to prevent various cancers, including breast cancer [17]. On the other hand, high energy intake is significantly related to breast risk, so adherence to healthier dietary patterns seems to affect disease risk [17]. Moreover, high consumption of red meat, animal fat, and refined carbohydrates leads to an increased risk of breast cancer [17, 20]. In contrast, adhering to a healthy dietary pattern, including increasing the consumption of fruits, vegetables, whole grains, and dietary fiber, is associated with a reduction in the risk of breast cancer [17, 21–23]. Since the results obtained from studies based on the measurement of the relationship between specific foods and nutrients are inconsistent, the analysis of food patterns as a common ancillary method to investigate the relationship between diet and disease risk has received much attention from researchers [24, 25].

Only a few studies have evaluated the relationship between dietary patterns and breast cancer [26–29]. According to epidemiological findings, both Western and prudent dietary patterns are related to the prognosis of breast cancer [26, 27].

The findings obtained from two recent systematic review studies have shown that adherence to a prudent or healthy dietary pattern is related to reducing the risk of breast cancer [21, 24, 30]. In addition, Zhang et al. reported that a dietary pattern rich in fruits, vegetables, and soybeans leads to a reduction in the risk of breast cancer [31].

Recently, instead of using specific foods as indicators of dietary intake and nutritional status, component food group analysis has been used to determine dietary patterns [32]. According to the findings, adherence to a dietary pattern with a higher content of plant-based diet and less content of animal-based foods is associated with reducing the risk of chronic disorders and ultimately mortality [32]. However, the general public's adherence to the vegetarian or vegan diet due to the restrictions may not be accurate and comprehensive. While there may be more adherence to the pro-vegetarian dietary pattern (PDP) due to the reduction of restrictions, including reducing the consumption of animal-based foods instead of eliminating animal products [32]. However, little evidence of the relationship between a plant-based diet and breast cancer incidence has been reported [32–34].

According to recent findings, adherence to a healthy plant-based diet has been associated with a reduction in the incidence of breast cancer, especially for tumors that become aggressive [33]. In a large prospective cohort study on 10,812 women in the Seguimiento Universidad de Navarra (SUN) project, which is a Spanish study, Romanos-Nonclares et al. in 2020 showed that moderate adherence to a vegetarian diet may reduce the risk of breast cancer [34]. In a population-based case-control study on women aged >30 years in Isfahan, Iran, between July 2013 and July 2015 conducted by Rigi et al., it has been shown that in Iranian women, greater adherence to an overall plant-based diet and a healthy plant-based diet is associated with a decrease in the risk of breast cancer, while more adherence to an unhealthy plant-based diet is associated with an increase in the risk of breast cancer [35]. In the study by Rigi et al. [35], the overall plant-based diet index (PDI) based on the algorithm developed by Martinez-Gonzalez et al. [36] and two versions of the healthy plant-based diet index (hPDI) and unhealthy plant-based diet index (uPDI) proposed by Satija et al. [37] have been evaluated.

Category of healthy plant food groups includes whole grains, fruits, vegetables, nuts, legumes, and vegetable oil, and less healthy plant food groups include fruit juice, sugar-sweetened beverages, refined grains, and potatoes, as well as animal food groups, which include a wide range of animal fats, dairy, eggs, fish/seafood, red meat, poultry, and miscellaneous animal-based foods [35, 38–43]. In another case-control study in Iranian women, it was also shown that adherence to the PDP is associated with a decreased chance of developing breast cancer [32]. In this study, to calculate PDP, two categories of plant-based food groups including vegetables, fruits, cereals, legumes, potatoes, olive oil, and nuts, as well as animal-based food groups including animal fats, fish, dairy products, eggs, and meat products, were evaluated [32]. The overall score of PDP is determined between 12 (minimum adherence) and 60 (maximum adherence) [32].

In the PDI and hPDI, scores of 10 and 1 correspond to the highest and lowest consumption of plant foods and healthy plant foods, respectively. Also, in uPDI, scores of 10 and 1 are attributed to the maximum and minimum consumption of unhealthy plant foods, respectively. To determine each of the PDI, hPDI, and uPDI indices, the scores are finally added up and a total score is obtained in the range of 18 to 180, where a higher score is associated with greater adherence to the dietary pattern (228–230).

## 5. Vegetarian diet and breast cancer

Although, the findings are insufficient to evaluate the relationship between diet and breast cancer risk [44], a reduction in breast cancer risk has been reported following an increase in fruit and vegetable consumption [21, 44–47]. In this regard, this effect has been investigated for postmenopausal and premenopausal breast cancer, as well as particular hormone receptor variants of breast cancer [44]. Since postmenopausal breast cancer is more influenced by lifestyle and environmental factors, this relationship was considered stronger for this group of patients [44]. Meanwhile, a strong relationship between adherence to a prudent diet pattern and premenopausal breast cancer has also been reported [44]. Additionally, a protective effect of higher fruit and vegetable consumption has also been shown for ER breast cancer risk [44].

Rizzo et al. [48] and Orlich et al. [49] have reported that vegans have more physical activity, consume fewer energy-dense nutrients, less sodium, and dairy and animal proteins. They also have a higher consumption of fiber-rich foods, vitamins, and vegetable proteins such as fruits and vegetables, whole grains, nuts, and soybeans. Additionally, they have a history of consuming less alcohol [44]. In this regard, Catsburg et al. [50] showed that individuals who follow all recommendations have a 31% lower risk of breast cancer than those who follow only one of them.

In a case-control study on 134 women with breast cancer and 265 without cancer (control) who were chosen from the two referral hospitals (Imam Hossein and Shohadaye Tajrish hospitals) in Tehran City (convenient sampling from September 2015 to February 2016), Hosseini et al. reported that greater adherence to the PDP in Iranian women is associated with a lower chance of developing breast cancer [32]. In addition, they showed that a diet rich in plant-based foods and poor in dairy products is associated with reducing the risk of breast cancer, especially in postmenopausal women [32]. Similarly, in the case-control study on 233 breast cancer patients and 236 age-matched controls in the surgical department of Taipei Tzu Chi Hospital, Chang et al. have emphasized the protective role of a vegetarian diet as an example of a plant-based diet against the risk of breast cancer [51]. Other studies have also indicated an inverse relationship between a higher score for greater adherence to a plant-based diet and a reduction in the risk of breast cancer [32, 33, 35, 51–53].

The term "vegetarian diet" is used to describe a special dietary pattern that avoids the consumption of meat fat and processed meat [51]. As dos Santos et al. showed in a population-based case-control study among South Asian migrant women from the Indian subcontinent resident in England, lifelong vegetarianism may have a protective effect against breast cancer due to its higher content of vegetables and pulses [54]. In another study on 69,120 participants of the Adventist Health Study-2, Tantamango-Bartley et al. reported that a lower risk of breast cancer in vegans is possible [55]. Cade et al. also showed in the United Kingdom Women's Cohort Study (UKWCS) on 35,372 women aged between 35 to 69 years, who were recruited from 1995 to 1998, that adherence to a vegetarian diet pattern is associated with a 12% reduction in the risk of breast cancer, although this relationship was not statistically significant [56].

Comprehensive and complete information is not available to explain the inverse relationship between the vegetarian dietary pattern and breast cancer [51]. However, adherence to vegetarian and vegan dietary patterns is associated with an increase in the consumption of plant-based foods and a decrease in the consumption of red meat and processed meat, which helps to reach an ideal weight [51]. Evidence for comparing vegetarian and nonvegetarian groups is limited [51]. However, it has been shown that vegans have a lower body mass index (BMI) than nonvegetarians, but no significant difference was observed in their functional immunocompetence [51]. Moreover, there was no significant difference between the levels of estradiol and testosterone between the two vegetarian and nonvegetarian groups [51]. However, Chang et al. reported that vegetarians have a higher daily intake of soy isoflavones than nonvegetarians [51]. The relationship between soy isoflavone consumption and reduced breast cancer risk has also been shown [51, 57]. Thus, the protective role of soy isoflavone consumption against breast cancer has been suggested [51].

Isoflavones are the major phytoestrogens found in soybean products that interact with alpha and beta ERs and may act as estrogen mimics and regulate estrogen levels [51]. Isoflavones act as weak estrogens when the level of estrogen in the body is low, and when the level of estrogen in the body is high, they inhibit the function of estrogen [51]. In this view, vegetarians and vegans who regularly consume soy have higher serum isoflavone levels [51, 58]. Therefore, these findings support the possible chemo-preventive role of isoflavones [51]. Additionally, the antiproliferative, proapoptotic, antiangiogenic, antioxidant, and anti-inflammatory properties of soy have also been proposed [44, 59]. Among other possible protective mechanisms of the vegetarian dietary pattern against cancer, it can be mentioned an increase in the consumption of fruits and vegetables [51].

In general, it has been shown that the relationship between a plant-based diet and breast cancer risk may be related to a higher intake of healthy plant products, including fruits, vegetables, legumes, and whole grains, along with a higher intake of fiber and micronutrients such as vitamin C, vitamin E, folate, carotenoids, and trace minerals including selenium, zinc, copper, and manganese. Additionally, many non-nutrients such as phytoestrogens, phenolic acid, lignan, and carotenoids affect cellular differentiation and apoptosis [35]. Dietary folate affects the expression of critical tumor suppressors and proto-oncogenes due to its role in DNA methylation [35].

Dietary fiber also has estrogen-modulatory effects, as well as removing damaged cells from the digestive tract, and bile acids, and, as a result, reducing cell proliferation and the possibility of mutations. It also reduces N-nitroso compounds, increases immunity, and produces anti-inflammatory cytokines involved in the initiation and progression of mammary cell growth [35]. It may have a protective effect against the risk of cancer through these properties [35].

The anticancer properties of phytoestrogens, phenolic acid, and lignan have also been suggested due to their modulating effect on the hormonal pathway through antioxidant, antiproliferative, antiangiogenic, and apoptotic properties [35, 60]. Among other features of the vegan diet, a higher intake of nonessential amino acids has been mentioned, which has led to regulation of the insulin-glucagon axis [44, 61–63], resulting in greater tissue sensitivity to insulin and a decrease in liver production and serum levels of insulin-like growth factor 1 (IGF-1) [44]. The relationship between the increased level of IGF-1 and the progression of several cancers as well as its mitogenic, antiapoptotic, and angiogenic effects have been shown, especially in mammary cell lines [35, 64, 65].

## 6. Conclusions

In sum, based on these findings, it seems that vegetarian diets may have a potential role in alleviating the development and progression of breast cancer through their several anticancer properties. However, more studies are suggested to investigate the clear and comprehensive mechanism by comparing the effect of a vegetarian diet and a nonvegetarian diet on breast cancer risk in premenopausal and postmenopausal women.

## Author details

Pegah Hadi Sichani[1], Maede Makhtoomi[2,3], Masoud Amini Kahrizsangi[4], Zainab Shateri[5], Mehran Nouri[6]* and Marzieh Mahmoodi[2,7]*

1 Department of Community Nutrition, School of Nutrition and Food Sciences, Nutrition and Food Security Research Center, Students' Research Committee, Isfahan University of Medical Sciences, Isfahan, Iran

2 Student Research Committee, Shiraz University of Medical Sciences, Shiraz, Iran

3 Health Policy Research Center, Institute of Health, Shiraz University of Medical Sciences, Shiraz, Iran

4 Department of Community Nutrition, School of Nutrition and Food Sciences, Isfahan University of Medical Sciences, Isfahan, Iran

5 Department of Nutrition and Biochemistry, School of Medicine, Ilam University of Medical Sciences, Ilam, Iran

6 Cancer Research Center, Health Research Institute, Babol University of Medical Sciences, Babol, Iran

7 Department of Clinical Nutrition, School of Nutrition and Food Science, Shiraz University of Medical Sciences, Shiraz, Iran

*Address all correspondence to: mehran_nouri71@yahoo.com
and marzieh.mahmoodi@gmail.com

## References

[1] Zamzam S et al. Dietary patterns associated with breast cancer in the Middle East: A scoping review. Nutrients. 2024;**16**(5):579

[2] Momenimovahed Z, Salehiniya H. Epidemiological characteristics of and risk factors for breast cancer in the world. Breast Cancer (Dove Med Press). 2019;**11**:151-164

[3] Onitilo AA et al. Breast cancer subtypes based on ER/PR and Her2 expression: Comparison of clinicopathologic features and survival. Clinical Medicine & Research. 2009;7(1-2):4-13

[4] Smolarz B, Nowak AZ, Romanowicz H. Breast cancer-epidemiology, classification, pathogenesis and treatment (review of literature). Cancers (Basel). 2022;**14**(10):2569

[5] Hortobagyi GN et al. The global breast cancer burden: Variations in epidemiology and survival. Clinical Breast Cancer. 2005;**6**(5):391-401

[6] Youlden DR et al. Incidence and mortality of female breast cancer in the Asia-Pacific region. Cancer Biology & Medicine. 2014;**11**(2):101-115

[7] Ghoncheh M et al. Epidemiology, incidence and mortality of breast cancer in Asia. Asian Pacific Journal of Cancer Prevention. 2016;**17**(S3):47-52

[8] Pourhabibi-Zarandi F et al. Dietary quality index and the risk of breast cancer: A case-control study. BMC Women's Health. 2023;**23**(1):469

[9] Haghighat S, Omidi Z, Ghanbari-Motlagh A. Trend of breast cancer incidence in Iran during a fifteen-year interval according to National Cancer Registry Reports. Iranian-Journal of-Breast-Diseases. 2022;**15**(2):4-17

[10] Roshandel G et al. Cancer in Iran 2008 to 2025: Recent incidence trends and short-term predictions of the future burden. International Journal of Cancer. 2021;**149**(3):594-605

[11] Kamińska M et al. Breast cancer risk factors. Przeglad Menopauzalny. 2015;**14**(3):196-202

[12] De Cicco P et al. Nutrition and breast cancer: A literature review on prevention, treatment and recurrence. Nutrients. 2019;**11**(7):1514

[13] Nouri M et al. Effect of serum lipid profile on the risk of breast cancer: Systematic review and meta-analysis of 1,628,871 women. Journal of Clinical Medicine. 2022;**11**(15):4503

[14] Giles ED et al. Obesity and overfeeding affecting both tumor and systemic metabolism activates the progesterone receptor to contribute to postmenopausal breast cancer. Cancer Research. 2012;**72**(24):6490-6501

[15] Mourouti N et al. Diet and breast cancer: A systematic review. International Journal of Food Sciences and Nutrition. 2015;**66**(1):1-42

[16] Jacobs I et al. Dietary patterns and breast cancer risk in black urban south African women: The SABC study. Nutrients. 2021;**13**(11):4106

[17] Fentie H, Ntenda PAM, Tiruneh FN. Dietary pattern and other factors of breast cancer among women: A case control study in Northwest Ethiopia. BMC Cancer. 2023;**23**(1):1050

[18] Shams-White MM et al. Operationalizing the 2018 World Cancer Research Fund/American Institute for Cancer Research (WCRF/AICR) cancer prevention recommendations: A standardized scoring system. Nutrients. 2019;**11**(7):1572

[19] Wild C, Weiderpass E, Stewart BW. World cancer report: cancer research for cancer prevention. 2020: International Agency for Research on Cancer

[20] Cho E et al. Red meat intake and risk of breast cancer among premenopausal women. Archives of Internal Medicine. 2006;**166**(20):2253-2259

[21] Brennan SF et al. Dietary patterns and breast cancer risk: A systematic review and meta-analysis. The American Journal of Clinical Nutrition. 2010;**91**(5):1294-1302

[22] Dong JY et al. Dietary fiber intake and risk of breast cancer: A meta-analysis of prospective cohort studies. The American Journal of Clinical Nutrition. 2011;**94**(3):900-905

[23] Malin AS et al. Intake of fruits, vegetables and selected micronutrients in relation to the risk of breast cancer. International Journal of Cancer. 2003;**105**(3):413-418

[24] Baglietto L et al. Dietary patterns and risk of breast cancer. British Journal of Cancer. 2011;**104**(3):524-531

[25] Lee JY, Cho HI, Kimm H. Dietary Patterns and Breast Cancer Risk: A KCPS-II Cohort Study. European Journal of Breast Health. 2021;**20**(4):262-269

[26] Kim N-H et al. Dietary pattern and health-related quality of life among breast cancer survivors. BMC Women's Health. 2018;**18**(1):65

[27] Kroenke CH et al. Dietary patterns and survival after breast cancer diagnosis. Journal of Clinical Oncology. 2005;**23**(36):9295-9303

[28] Kwan ML et al. Dietary patterns and breast cancer recurrence and survival among women with early-stage breast cancer. Journal of Clinical Oncology. 2009;**27**(6):919-926

[29] Vrieling A et al. Dietary patterns and survival in German postmenopausal breast cancer survivors. British Journal of Cancer. 2013;**108**(1):188-192

[30] Edefonti V et al. Dietary patterns and breast cancer: A review with focus on methodological issues. Nutrition Reviews. 2009;**67**(6):297-314

[31] Zhang CX et al. Dietary patterns and breast cancer risk among Chinese women. Cancer Causes & Control. 2011;**22**(1):115-124

[32] Hosseini Y et al. Pro-vegetarian dietary pattern and risk of breast cancer: A case-control study. Breast Cancer Research and Treatment. 2024;**205**(2):395-402

[33] Romanos-Nanclares A et al. Healthful and unhealthful plant-based diets and risk of breast cancer in U.S. women: Results from the Nurses' health studies. Cancer Epidemiology, Biomarkers & Prevention. 2021;**30**(10):1921-1931

[34] Romanos-Nanclares A et al. Healthful and unhealthful provegetarian food patterns and the incidence of breast cancer: Results from a Mediterranean cohort. Nutrition. 2020;**79-80**:110884

[35] Rigi S et al. The association between plant-based dietary patterns and risk of breast cancer: A case-control study. Scientific Reports. 2021;**11**(1):3391

[36] Martínez-González MA et al. A provegetarian food pattern and reduction in total mortality in the Prevención con Dieta Mediterránea (PREDIMED) study. The American Journal of Clinical Nutrition. 2014;**100**(Suppl. 1):320s-328s

[37] Satija A et al. Plant-based dietary patterns and incidence of type 2 diabetes in US men and women: Results from three prospective cohort studies. PLoS Medicine. 2016;**13**(6):e1002039

[38] Ghadiri M et al. Healthy plant-based diet index as a determinant of bone mineral density in osteoporotic postmenopausal women: A case-control study. Frontiers in Nutrition. 2022;**9**:1083685

[39] Lotfi M et al. Plant-based diets could ameliorate the risk factors of cardiovascular diseases in adults with chronic diseases. Food Science & Nutrition. 2023;**11**(3):1297-1308

[40] Nouri M et al. The relationship between plant-based diet index and semen parameters of men with infertility: A cross-sectional study. International Journal of Fertility and Sterility. 2022;**16**(4):310-319

[41] Zare M et al. Effect of a plant-based diet on oxidative stress biomarkers in male footballers. Scientific Reports. 2024;**14**(1):3700

[42] Borazjani M et al. Association of plant-based diets with lipid profile and anthropometric indices: A cross-sectional study. Nutrition & Food Science. 2022;**52**(5):830-842

[43] Jafari F et al. Association of plant-based dietary patterns with metabolic syndrome: Baseline results from the Persian Kavar cohort study (PKCS). International Journal of Food Sciences and Nutrition. 2023;**74**(2):291-301

[44] Penniecook-Sawyers JA et al. Vegetarian dietary patterns and the risk of breast cancer in a low-risk population. The British Journal of Nutrition. 2016;**115**(10):1790-1797

[45] Butler LM et al. A vegetable-fruit-soy dietary pattern protects against breast cancer among postmenopausal Singapore Chinese women. The American Journal of Clinical Nutrition. 2010;**91**(4):1013-1019

[46] Cottet V et al. Postmenopausal breast cancer risk and dietary patterns in the E3N-EPIC prospective cohort study. American Journal of Epidemiology. 2009;**170**(10):1257-1267

[47] Wu AH et al. Dietary patterns and breast cancer risk in Asian American women. The American Journal of Clinical Nutrition. 2009;**89**(4):1145-1154

[48] Rizzo NS et al. Nutrient profiles of vegetarian and nonvegetarian dietary patterns. Journal of the Academy of Nutrition and Dietetics. 2013;**113**(12):1610-1619

[49] Orlich MJ et al. Patterns of food consumption among vegetarians and non-vegetarians. The British Journal of Nutrition. 2014;**112**(10):1644-1653

[50] Catsburg C, Miller AB, Rohan TE. Adherence to cancer prevention guidelines and risk of breast cancer. International Journal of Cancer. 2014;**135**(10):2444-2452

[51] Chang YJ et al. Is vegetarian diet associated with a lower risk of breast cancer in Taiwanese women? BMC Public Health. 2017;**17**(1):800

[52] Catsburg C et al. Dietary patterns and breast cancer risk: A study in 2 cohorts. The American Journal of Clinical Nutrition. 2015;**101**(4):817-823

[53] Link LB et al. Dietary patterns and breast cancer risk in the California teachers study cohort. The American Journal of Clinical Nutrition. 2013;**98**(6):1524-1532

[54] Dos Santos Silva I et al. Lifelong vegetarianism and risk of breast cancer: A population-based case-control study among South Asian migrant women living in England. International Journal of Cancer. 2002;**99**(2):238-244

[55] Tantamango-Bartley Y et al. Vegetarian diets and the incidence of cancer in a low-risk population. Cancer Epidemiology, Biomarkers & Prevention. 2013;**22**(2):286-294

[56] Cade JE et al. Common dietary patterns and risk of breast cancer: Analysis from the United Kingdom Women's cohort study. Nutrition and Cancer. 2010;**62**(3):300-306

[57] Yamamoto S et al. Soy, isoflavones, and breast cancer risk in Japan. Journal of the National Cancer Institute. 2003;**95**(12):906-913

[58] Ko KP et al. Plasma isoflavone concentration is associated with decreased risk of type 2 diabetes in Korean women but not men: Results from the Korean genome and epidemiology study. Diabetologia. 2015;**58**(4):726-735

[59] Wada K et al. Soy isoflavone intake and breast cancer risk in Japan: From the Takayama study. International Journal of Cancer. 2013;**133**(4):952-960

[60] Slavin JL. Mechanisms for the impact of whole grain foods on cancer risk. Journal of the American College of Nutrition. 2000;**19**(Suppl. 3):300s-307s

[61] McCarty MF. Vegan proteins may reduce risk of cancer, obesity, and cardiovascular disease by promoting increased glucagon activity. Medical Hypotheses. 1999;**53**(6):459-485

[62] McCarty MF. mTORC1 activity as a determinant of cancer risk--rationalizing the cancer-preventive effects of adiponectin, metformin, rapamycin, and low-protein vegan diets. Medical Hypotheses. 2011;**77**(4):642-648

[63] Clemmons DR, Underwood LE. Nutritional regulation of IGF-I and IGF binding proteins. Annual Review of Nutrition. 1991;**11**:393-412

[64] Muti P et al. Fasting glucose is a risk factor for breast cancer: A prospective study. Cancer Epidemiology, Biomarkers & Prevention. 2002;**11**(11):1361-1368

[65] Outwater JL, Nicholson A, Barnard N. Dairy products and breast cancer: The IGF-I, estrogen, and bGH hypothesis. Medical Hypotheses. 1997;**48**(6):453-461

Chapter 6

# Targeting Cancer Stem Cells in Gynecological Malignancies: Emerging Advanced Therapeutic Approaches

*Rama Satya Sri Kotipalli, Mani Sharma, Nemala Siva Kumar, Abhiram Kumar, Chhavi Dhiman, Mohini Rawat, Piyush Khandelia and Kumar Pranav Narayan*

**Abstract**

Cancer stem cells (CSCs) are a crucial subpopulation in gynecological tumors, defined by their self-renewal, differentiation potential, and resistance to conventional therapies. These cells are central to tumor initiation, progression, metastasis, and recurrence, making them key targets for innovative therapeutic strategies. This chapter will explore the molecular mechanisms that regulate CSCs, focusing on signaling pathways such as Wnt, Notch, and Hedgehog, which are critical for CSC maintenance and survival. It will also examine emerging therapeutic approaches aimed at eradicating CSCs, including pathway inhibitors, immune-based strategies, and combinatorial treatments. By targeting CSCs, these approaches hold the promise of overcoming resistance and achieving more reliable clinical responses in gynecological cancers. Further, this chapter delves into the challenges and future directions of translating CSC-targeted therapies into clinical practice.

**Keywords:** cancer stem cells (CSCs), gynecological malignancies, tumorigenesis, therapeutic resistance, targeted therapy, immunotherapy, tumor recurrence

## 1. Introduction

Introduction to cancer stem cells (CSCs): cancer stem cells (CSCs) are a unique subset of cells within tumors that possess the ability to self-renew and differentiate into diverse cell types, thereby sustaining tumor growth and heterogeneity [1]. First identified in hematological malignancies, the concept of CSCs has since expanded to encompass a variety of cancers, including gynecological malignancies. Unlike their differentiated counterparts, CSCs are capable of initiating tumor formation, leading to the hypothesis that these cells are responsible for tumor initiation, metastasis, and relapse after treatment. Their identification has reshaped our understanding of



IntechOpen

cancer biology, shifting the focus from a purely cellular perspective to a more nuanced view that considers the hierarchical organization of tumors [2].

### 1.1 Characteristics of CSCs

One of the defining features of CSCs is their self-renewal capability, which enables them to undergo numerous rounds of division while maintaining the undifferentiated state. This property is critical for the long-term persistence of the tumor, as CSCs can replenish the tumor cell population even after aggressive treatments that target bulk tumor cells. Additionally, CSCs demonstrate significant differentiation potential, allowing them to give rise to a heterogeneous population of tumor cells, which may exhibit varying degrees of sensitivity to therapies. This heterogeneity complicates treatment strategies and contributes to the challenges of eradicating tumors completely [3].

Another hallmark of CSCs is their inherent resistance to conventional therapies, such as chemotherapy and radiation. This resistance is attributed to several factors, including the expression of drug efflux pumps, enhanced DNA repair mechanisms, and the ability to enter a quiescent state, making them less susceptible to treatments designed to target rapidly dividing cells. Consequently, the presence of CSCs in tumors is often linked to treatment failure and disease recurrence, emphasizing their role as a critical target for innovative therapeutic approaches [4].

Furthermore, CSCs are characterized by specific surface markers that distinguish them from non-stem cancer cells. Markers such as CD44, CD133, and ALDH1 are commonly used to identify and isolate CSCs, facilitating research into their biology and therapeutic targeting. Understanding the molecular pathways and signaling networks that regulate these cells, such as the Wnt, Notch, and Hedgehog pathways, is crucial for developing effective strategies aimed at eliminating CSCs and improving treatment outcomes in gynecological cancers. As research continues to uncover the complexities of CSCs, it becomes increasingly clear that targeting these cells is essential for achieving lasting remission and improving patient survival rates [5].

### 1.2 Role of CSCs in gynecological tumors

CSCs play a pivotal role in the biology of gynecological tumors, significantly influencing tumor initiation, progression, and metastasis. In cancers such as ovarian, endometrial, and cervical cancers, CSCs are often implicated in the early stages of tumor development. Their ability to self-renew and differentiate contributes to the establishment of a diverse tumor microenvironment, which can promote tumor aggressiveness and heterogeneity. This diversity is critical as it enables the tumor to adapt to therapeutic pressures and evade treatment, resulting in relapses and metastasis. CSCs' presence often correlates with poor prognostic outcomes, making them key targets for therapeutic intervention [6].

Moreover, CSCs in gynecological tumors exhibit unique molecular signatures and signaling pathways that differentiate them from non-stem cancer cells. For instance, alterations in the Wnt, Notch, and Hedgehog signaling pathways have been shown to regulate the maintenance and proliferation of CSCs, contributing to tumor survival and resistance to therapies. These pathways not only enhance the self-renewal capabilities of CSCs but also influence their differentiation potential, thereby affecting the overall tumor behavior. Additionally, CSCs can secrete factors that create a favorable niche for tumor growth and support the recruitment of stromal cells, further complicating the treatment landscape [7].

The role of CSCs extends beyond tumor biology; they are also integral to the mechanisms of metastasis in gynecological cancers. CSCs possess enhanced migratory and invasive properties, facilitating the spread of cancer to distant sites. Their ability to survive in the bloodstream and adapt to the foreign microenvironment is crucial for successful metastasis. Understanding the multifaceted role of CSCs in gynecological tumors is essential for developing targeted therapies that can effectively eliminate these cells, thereby improving patient outcomes and reducing the likelihood of recurrence. Addressing the challenges posed by CSCs will be key in advancing treatment strategies and enhancing the efficacy of current interventions in gynecological oncology [8].

## 2. Molecular mechanisms regulating CSCs

### 2.1 Overview of key signaling pathways

The regulation of CSCs is intricately controlled by various molecular signaling pathways that govern their self-renewal, differentiation, and survival. Among these, the Wnt, Notch, and Hedgehog pathways are pivotal in maintaining CSC properties and driving tumor progression. These pathways interact with each other and with the tumor microenvironment, forming a complex network that influences CSC behavior. Disruptions or aberrations in these signaling cascades can lead to the activation of CSCs, contributing to tumor heterogeneity and resistance to conventional therapies. Understanding these pathways is essential for devising targeted therapies aimed at eradicating CSCs and improving patient outcomes in gynecological malignancies [9].

#### *2.1.1 Wnt pathway*

The Wnt signaling pathway is critically involved in the regulation of CSCs, particularly in gynecological tumors. This pathway is activated by the binding of Wnt proteins to Frizzled receptors, leading to the stabilization and accumulation of β-catenin in the cytoplasm and its subsequent translocation to the nucleus. Once in the nucleus, β-catenin forms a complex with TCF/LEF transcription factors, activating the transcription of target genes that promote cell proliferation, self-renewal, and pluripotency. In CSCs, the Wnt pathway is often upregulated, supporting their capacity for self-renewal and contributing to tumorigenicity [10].

In gynecological cancers, aberrant activation of the Wnt pathway has been linked to poor prognosis and treatment resistance. For instance, studies have shown that high levels of β-catenin are associated with aggressive tumor phenotypes and increased CSC populations in ovarian and endometrial cancers. Targeting the Wnt signaling pathway holds promise for therapeutic strategies aimed at reducing the CSC pool, thereby enhancing the efficacy of existing treatments. Inhibitors of Wnt signaling are currently being investigated in preclinical and clinical settings, emphasizing the need for further exploration of this pathway's role in the maintenance of CSCs and its potential as a therapeutic target in gynecological malignancies [11].

Agents like IWP-2 and XAV939 are being tested in preclinical studies for their ability to reduce CSC populations in ovarian cancer. While specific clinical trials are limited, combining Wnt inhibitors with chemotherapy shows potential [12].

### 2.1.2 Notch pathway

The Notch signaling pathway plays a crucial role in regulating CSCs, influencing their self-renewal, differentiation, and tumorigenic potential. Notch signaling is initiated when Notch receptors on the surface of a cell bind to ligands presented by adjacent cells, leading to the cleavage of the Notch receptor and the release of the Notch intracellular domain (NICD). This NICD then translocates to the nucleus, where it interacts with transcriptional coactivators to modulate the expression of target genes involved in cell fate determination. In the context of CSCs, Notch signaling promotes the maintenance of stem-like properties, thus sustaining the CSC pool within tumors [13].

In gynecological cancers, such as ovarian and cervical tumors, the activation of the Notch pathway has been implicated in enhancing the aggressiveness of tumors and their resistance to conventional therapies. High levels of Notch signaling activity are often associated with increased CSC populations, leading to enhanced tumor growth and metastasis. Furthermore, Notch signaling has been shown to interact with other pathways, such as Wnt and Hedgehog, creating a complex regulatory network that further supports CSC survival and proliferation [14].

Targeting the Notch pathway presents a promising strategy for CSC-directed therapies in gynecological malignancies. Various approaches, including small molecule inhibitors and monoclonal antibodies targeting Notch receptors or ligands, are under investigation. By inhibiting Notch signaling, it may be possible to reduce the CSC population, enhance the effectiveness of existing treatments, and ultimately improve clinical outcomes for patients. The continued exploration of the Notch pathway's role in CSC biology is essential for the development of innovative therapeutic strategies that address the challenges posed by these resilient cells [15].

γ-Secretase inhibitors such as LY411575 and DAPT are under investigation, demonstrating efficacy in reducing tumor growth in early-phase trials. Ongoing studies are exploring their use alongside standard treatments in recurrent ovarian cancer [16].

### 2.1.3 Hedgehog pathway

The Hedgehog (Hh) signaling pathway is a critical regulator of cell growth, differentiation, and tissue patterning during embryonic development. In the context of cancer, particularly in gynecological malignancies, the Hedgehog pathway has been shown to play a significant role in the maintenance and function of CSCs. Activation of this pathway occurs when Hedgehog ligands bind to Patched (Ptch) receptors, relieving the inhibition on Smoothened (Smo), a key transducer of the signal. This leads to the activation of downstream transcription factors, including Gli proteins, which promote the expression of target genes involved in cell proliferation, survival, and self-renewal [17].

In gynecological tumors, aberrant activation of the Hedgehog pathway has been associated with tumor progression and metastasis. Research has demonstrated that CSCs in ovarian and endometrial cancers exhibit heightened Hedgehog signaling activity, which contributes to their stem-like properties and resistance to chemotherapy. This pathway not only supports the CSC population but also enhances the tumor's ability to invade surrounding tissues and establish secondary growths. Additionally, the interaction of Hedgehog signaling with other pathways, such as Wnt and Notch, further complicates the regulatory networks that govern CSC behavior [18].

Targeting the Hedgehog pathway offers a promising therapeutic strategy for combating CSCs in gynecological cancers. Inhibitors of the Hedgehog signaling cascade, such as vismodegib and sonidegib, are being explored in clinical trials, demonstrating potential in reducing tumor growth and improving patient outcomes. By effectively disrupting Hedgehog signaling, it may be possible to decrease the CSC population, enhance sensitivity to conventional therapies, and ultimately lead to more durable responses in gynecological cancer treatment. Continued research into the mechanisms of Hedgehog signaling in CSCs is essential for developing innovative approaches to target these resilient cells and improve therapeutic efficacy [19].

Vismodegib and sonidegib, initially developed for basal cell carcinoma, are being tested in gynecological cancers. Clinical trials have shown they can reduce tumor size and improve responses, particularly in ovarian and endometrial cancers [20].

### 2.2 Interactions between pathways and CSC maintenance

The maintenance of CSCs is not solely governed by individual signaling pathways but is significantly influenced by the intricate interactions among various pathways, such as Wnt, Notch, and Hedgehog. These pathways often converge to regulate key aspects of CSC biology, including self-renewal, differentiation, and tumorigenicity. For instance, cross-talk between the Wnt and Notch pathways has been observed, where the activation of one can enhance the signaling of the other, creating a supportive microenvironment for CSCs. This synergy can lead to a more aggressive tumor phenotype and contribute to therapeutic resistance, as CSCs leverage multiple signaling networks to adapt to treatment pressures [21].

Furthermore, the Hedgehog pathway also interacts with Wnt and Notch signaling, providing a multifaceted regulatory framework that sustains CSC populations in gynecological cancers. Research indicates that Hedgehog signaling can upregulate Notch activity, promoting the maintenance of stem-like characteristics within tumors. This interconnected signaling not only supports the survival and self-renewal of CSCs but also facilitates their capacity for differentiation into various tumor cell types, thereby enhancing tumor heterogeneity. Such plasticity is a hallmark of CSCs, making them particularly challenging targets for conventional therapies [22].

Understanding the interactions between these pathways is crucial for developing effective therapeutic strategies aimed at eradicating CSCs. By targeting multiple signaling networks simultaneously, it may be possible to disrupt the intricate support system that sustains CSCs, leading to improved treatment responses. Investigational therapies that incorporate inhibitors of Wnt, Notch, and Hedgehog pathways are being studied, with the goal of overcoming the resistance mechanisms that CSCs employ. Continued research into the complex interplay of these pathways will be essential for advancing personalized treatment approaches and improving outcomes for patients with gynecological malignancies [20].

## 3. Emerging therapeutic approaches

### 3.1 Pathway inhibitors

Targeting Wnt, Notch, and Hedgehog: The development of targeted therapies that inhibit key signaling pathways—namely Wnt, Notch, and Hedgehog—has emerged as a promising strategy for addressing the challenges posed by CSCs in gynecological malignancies. These pathways are critically involved in the maintenance and proliferation of CSCs, and their dysregulation is often associated with tumor progression and treatment resistance. By inhibiting these pathways, therapeutic agents aim to reduce the CSC population, enhance the efficacy of existing treatments, and ultimately improve patient outcomes [23].

Wnt pathway inhibitors, such as ICG-001 and LGK974, have shown potential in preclinical studies by disrupting the Wnt signaling cascade that is often hyperactivated in various cancers, including ovarian and endometrial tumors. By targeting β-catenin, a central player in the Wnt pathway, these inhibitors can hinder CSC self-renewal and promote differentiation of these cells into more mature, nontumorigenic cell types. Similarly, Notch inhibitors like gamma-secretase inhibitors (GSIs) have been explored for their ability to block Notch signaling, thereby disrupting the maintenance of CSCs and enhancing sensitivity to conventional therapies. This is particularly relevant in gynecological cancers, where Notch signaling has been implicated in tumor aggressiveness and recurrence [24].

Clinical trials exploring combinations of γ-secretase inhibitors (e.g., DAPT) with Wnt inhibitors like XAV939 show promise in reducing tumor growth and CSC populations in ovarian cancer.

The Hedgehog signaling pathway also presents a critical target for CSC-directed therapies. Inhibitors such as vismodegib and sonidegib have been developed to block Smoothened (Smo), a key component of the Hedgehog pathway. These agents have demonstrated efficacy in preclinical models, leading to decreased CSC populations and reduced tumor growth. The combinatorial use of pathway inhibitors alongside traditional therapies may hold significant promise, as it can potentially overcome the adaptive resistance mechanisms employed by CSCs. Continued research into these emerging therapeutic approaches is essential for optimizing treatment regimens that specifically target the unique biology of CSCs, ultimately contributing to more effective management of gynecological cancers [25].

Vismodegib is being investigated alongside Wnt pathway inhibitors, demonstrating potential in enhancing therapeutic responses and overcoming resistance in endometrial cancer models.

Triple pathway inhibition: Ongoing trials are assessing the safety and efficacy of combined therapies targeting Wnt, Notch, and Hedgehog pathways, aiming to improve patient outcomes by tackling CSCs from multiple angles [26].

### 3.2 Immune-based strategies

Cancer vaccines and immune checkpoint inhibitors: Emerging immune-based strategies have gained significant traction in the fight against gynecological malignancies, particularly those targeting CSCs. Cancer vaccines are designed to stimulate the immune system to recognize and attack tumor-associated antigens, including those expressed by CSCs. These vaccines can be peptide-based, dendritic cell-based, or whole-cell formulations, and their efficacy lies in their ability to generate a robust immune response specifically targeting CSC populations. For instance, personalized cancer vaccines that incorporate neoantigens—unique mutations found in an individual's tumor—show promise in enhancing the specificity of the immune response against CSCs, potentially leading to improved clinical outcomes and reduced recurrence rates [27].

In addition to cancer vaccines, immune checkpoint inhibitors represent another innovative approach to enhance the antitumor immune response. Agents such as pembrolizumab and nivolumab, which block programmed cell death protein 1 (PD-1) and its ligand PD-L1, have demonstrated significant efficacy in various cancers by reinvigorating T cell activity against tumor cells, including CSCs. Preclinical studies suggest that immune checkpoint inhibitors can effectively target the immunosuppressive microenvironment often associated with CSCs, overcoming their ability to evade immune surveillance. By enhancing T cell infiltration and promoting a more aggressive immune response against CSCs, these inhibitors hold the potential to complement existing therapies, potentially leading to more durable and effective treatment outcomes [28].

Combining cancer vaccines and immune checkpoint inhibitors could further augment therapeutic efficacy. Such combinatorial approaches can synergistically enhance the immune response by both priming the immune system through vaccination and removing inhibitory signals via checkpoint blockade. This multifaceted strategy aims to not only target the bulk tumor but also specifically eradicate CSCs, which are often responsible for treatment resistance and tumor relapse. Continued exploration of these immune-based strategies in clinical trials is essential for determining their effectiveness and optimizing their use in the context of gynecological cancers, paving the way for more effective and personalized therapeutic regimens [29].

### 3.3 Combinatorial treatments

Synergistic approaches to enhance efficacy: The complexity of cancer, particularly in gynecological malignancies, necessitates innovative treatment strategies that harness the strengths of multiple therapeutic modalities. Combinatorial treatments that integrate pathway inhibitors, immune-based therapies, and traditional chemotherapies are emerging as a powerful approach to enhance therapeutic efficacy and target CSCs. By strategically combining therapies, clinicians aim to exploit potential synergies, overcoming the inherent resistance mechanisms that CSCs often employ [30].

One promising avenue is the combination of immune checkpoint inhibitors with targeted therapies aimed at CSC pathways, such as Wnt or Notch signaling (**Figure 1**).

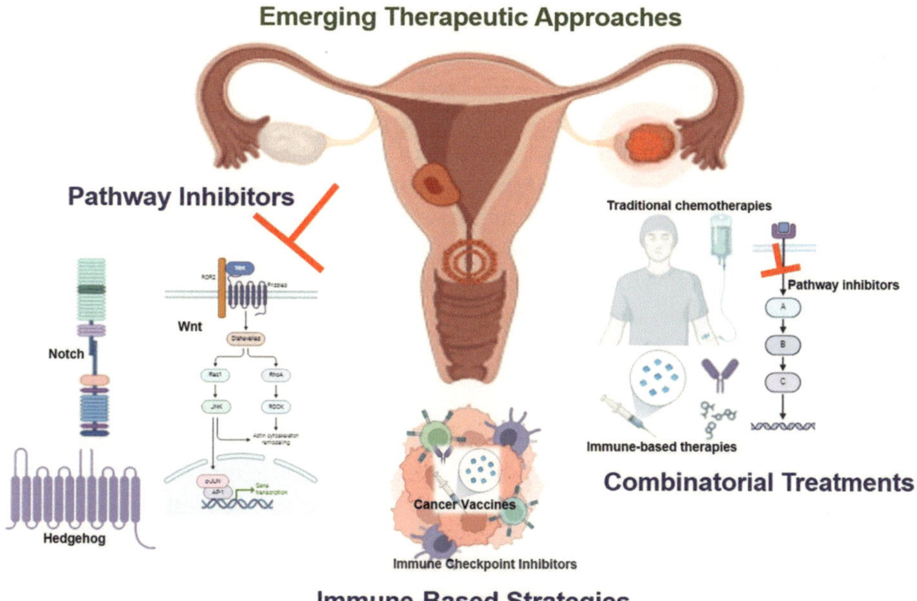


**Figure 1.**
*Emerging therapeutic approaches in gynecological malignancies.*

For example, using a Notch inhibitor alongside PD-1 blockade could simultaneously disrupt the survival pathways of CSCs while reinvigorating T cell responses against the tumor. This dual approach not only aims to reduce the CSC population but also enhances the overall immune response, potentially leading to more significant tumor regression and improved patient outcomes. Preclinical studies have shown that such combinations can lead to enhanced apoptosis in CSCs, thereby addressing one of the key challenges in treating gynecological cancers [31].

Furthermore, integrating chemotherapy with targeted therapies can create a robust treatment strategy that maximizes the impact on both the bulk tumor and the CSCs. For instance, chemotherapeutic agents can sensitize CSCs to pathway inhibitors, making them more vulnerable to treatment. By concurrently administering these therapies, oncologists can exploit the weaknesses in CSCs' protective mechanisms and promote more effective tumor eradication. The challenge lies in carefully designing treatment regimens that balance efficacy with potential toxicity, as the combined effects can lead to heightened side effects. Nonetheless, ongoing clinical trials are essential to elucidate the optimal combinations and sequences that will yield the best outcomes for patients with gynecological malignancies, marking a significant advancement in precision medicine approaches in oncology [32].

## 4. Clinical implications of targeting CSCs

### 4.1 Overcoming resistance to conventional therapies

Targeting CSCs presents a transformative opportunity to address one of the most pressing challenges in gynecological malignancies: the resistance to conventional therapies. CSCs are often responsible for tumor initiation, progression, and recurrence due to their unique properties, including self-renewal and differentiation potential. Traditional treatments, such as chemotherapy and radiation, primarily target rapidly dividing cells and may not effectively eradicate CSCs, which often exist in a quiescent state. This resistance can lead to treatment failure and relapse, underscoring the need for strategies that specifically target CSCs [33].

Emerging therapeutic approaches that focus on CSCs have the potential to enhance clinical outcomes by disrupting the pathways that confer their survival advantages. For instance, combining conventional therapies with agents that inhibit key signaling pathways—such as Wnt, Notch, and Hedgehog—can render CSCs more susceptible to cytotoxic effects. Studies have shown that when CSCs are simultaneously targeted alongside bulk tumor cells, there is a significant reduction in tumor recurrence and metastasis. This dual approach not only aims to eliminate existing tumors but also prevents the regeneration of the tumor from residual CSC populations, ultimately improving long-term patient survival rates [34].

Furthermore, targeting CSCs may facilitate the development of personalized treatment regimens tailored to the unique characteristics of an individual's tumor. By utilizing biomarkers to identify CSC populations and their specific vulnerabilities, oncologists can design targeted therapies that are more effective and less toxic than traditional approaches. This precision medicine strategy holds the promise of improving patient outcomes while minimizing adverse effects associated with conventional treatments. As research progresses, the integration of CSC-targeted therapies into clinical practice will be crucial for enhancing therapeutic efficacy, reducing recurrence rates, and ultimately transforming the landscape of treatment for gynecological cancers [23].

### 4.2 Enhancing clinical responses in gynecological cancers

Enhancing clinical responses in gynecological cancers requires a multifaceted approach that integrates innovative therapeutic strategies targeting the unique biology of these malignancies. One of the central tenets in this effort is the recognition of CSCs as pivotal players in tumor initiation, progression, and resistance to therapies. By focusing on the specific pathways that regulate CSCs—such as Wnt, Notch, and Hedgehog—researchers are developing targeted therapies that aim to eliminate these resilient cell populations. The efficacy of these approaches is further bolstered when combined with traditional treatments, leading to a more comprehensive attack on both the bulk tumor and its CSC component [35].

Clinical trials exploring the combination of CSC-targeting therapies with conventional chemotherapy and immunotherapy have shown promising results. For instance, the incorporation of immune checkpoint inhibitors alongside agents that inhibit CSC pathways has demonstrated enhanced antitumor immunity while directly targeting the CSCs responsible for relapse. This combinatorial approach not only improves initial clinical responses but also significantly reduces the likelihood of tumor recurrence, thereby enhancing overall survival rates. Such strategies emphasize the importance of personalized medicine, where treatment regimens are tailored based on the individual characteristics of the tumor and its CSC population.

Moreover, ongoing research into the molecular mechanisms governing CSC behavior is crucial for developing next-generation therapies that improve clinical outcomes in gynecological cancers. The identification of specific biomarkers associated with CSCs allows for more precise stratification of patients, enabling targeted interventions that are more effective and less toxic. As these innovative strategies are translated into clinical practice, they hold the potential to revolutionize the management of gynecological cancers, leading to improved patient outcomes and quality of life through a more effective and personalized treatment landscape [36].

#### *4.2.1 Cancer vaccines*

Personalized cancer vaccines: Trials are ongoing with neoantigen-based vaccines, such as the NeoVax platform, showing promise in eliciting strong immune responses specifically targeting CSCs in ovarian cancer patients.

Dendritic cell vaccines: Vaccines like sipuleucel-T are under investigation for cervical cancer, aiming to enhance T cell recognition of tumor-associated antigens.

#### *4.2.2 Immune checkpoint inhibitors*

Pembrolizumab and nivolumab: These PD-1 inhibitors have demonstrated efficacy in clinical settings, with ongoing studies assessing their impact on CSC populations in endometrial and ovarian cancers.

#### *4.2.3 Combination therapies*

Clinical trials are exploring the combination of checkpoint inhibitors with cancer vaccines, aiming to improve overall survival rates and minimize recurrence by targeting both the tumor and CSCs.

## 5. Challenges in translating CSC-targeted therapies to clinical practice

### 5.1 Identifying and isolating CSCs

Translating CSC-targeted therapies into clinical practice presents significant challenges, particularly in the identification and isolation of CSCs. CSCs are a rare subpopulation within tumors, and their unique properties—such as self-renewal, differentiation potential, and resistance to conventional therapies—make them difficult to characterize. Currently, there is no universally accepted marker or set of markers for accurately identifying CSCs across different gynecological malignancies. This lack of standardization complicates the isolation of these cells for research and therapeutic purposes, hindering the development of targeted therapies that effectively address their contributions to tumorigenesis and treatment resistance.

Moreover, the heterogeneity of CSCs within tumors poses additional challenges in accurately isolating and studying these cells. CSC populations can vary significantly between patients and even within the same tumor, reflecting a dynamic equilibrium influenced by the tumor microenvironment. This variability makes it difficult to establish consistent models for studying CSC biology and assessing the efficacy of targeted therapies. Additionally, the methodologies used for isolating CSCs—such as flow cytometry, magnetic-activated cell sorting, and sphere formation assays—can yield different results based on the techniques and markers employed. Therefore, there is an urgent need for innovative approaches and standardized protocols to better identify and isolate CSCs, ensuring that therapeutic strategies can be effectively translated from bench to bedside.

To address these challenges, collaborative efforts across disciplines are essential. Integrating insights from genomics, proteomics, and single-cell analysis can enhance our understanding of CSC characteristics and behaviors. Furthermore, the development of novel biomarkers that reliably distinguish CSCs from their differentiated counterparts will facilitate more accurate isolation and characterization. As researchers refine their ability to identify and isolate CSCs, the pathway to implementing effective CSC-targeted therapies in clinical practice will become clearer, ultimately leading to improved outcomes for patients with gynecological cancers.

#### *5.1.1 Biomarker development*

Research is ongoing to identify reliable biomarkers for CSCs, such as CD133 and ALDH1, although none are universally accepted across gynecological cancers. Clinical trials are testing these markers for efficacy in identifying CSC populations [37].

### 5.2 Isolation techniques

Innovative methodologies, like single-cell RNA sequencing and microfluidics, are being explored to enhance the precision of isolating CSCs. These approaches aim to overcome limitations of traditional methods like flow cytometry, which can yield inconsistent results.

#### *5.2.1 Collaborative research efforts*

Multidisciplinary studies are integrating genomics and proteomics to improve CSC characterization. For example, ongoing collaborations are focusing on refining protocols for isolating CSCs to facilitate the development of targeted therapies.

#### *5.2.1.1 Developing effective delivery systems*

The development of effective delivery systems for CSC-targeted therapies is critical for enhancing the therapeutic efficacy and specificity of treatment in gynecological cancers. Given the unique characteristics of CSCs, which often exhibit resistance to conventional therapies, traditional drug delivery methods may not adequately address the challenges posed by this cell population. Innovative delivery systems must be designed to effectively target CSCs while minimizing off-target effects on normal cells. One promising approach involves the use of nanotechnology, where nanoparticles can be engineered to encapsulate therapeutic agents specifically aimed at eradicating CSCs. These nanoparticles can be functionalized with ligands that bind to specific markers expressed on CSCs, thereby enhancing the precision of drug delivery and increasing the concentration of the therapeutic agent at the site of action.

Additionally, the choice of delivery route plays a crucial role in the effectiveness of CSC-targeted therapies. For instance, systemic delivery methods may require advanced formulations that ensure sustained release and controlled distribution of the drug, improving the chances of reaching CSCs in various tissue compartments. Alternatively, localized delivery systems—such as injectable hydrogels or implantable devices—offer the potential to deliver high concentrations of therapeutic agents directly to tumor sites, thereby reducing systemic toxicity and enhancing local efficacy. Combining these innovative delivery methods with CSC-targeted therapies can significantly improve patient outcomes by overcoming resistance mechanisms and achieving more reliable therapeutic responses.

The development of effective delivery systems also necessitates rigorous preclinical and clinical testing to evaluate their safety, efficacy, and optimal dosing regimens. Comprehensive studies examining the pharmacokinetics and biodistribution of these novel formulations will provide essential insights into their performance in vivo. Furthermore, collaboration among researchers, clinicians, and pharmaceutical developers is essential to facilitate the translation of these delivery systems from laboratory research to clinical applications. By prioritizing the development of targeted and effective delivery systems, the field can make significant strides toward overcoming the challenges associated with treating gynecological cancers, ultimately improving survival rates and quality of life for affected patients [38].

##### *5.2.1.1.1 Nanoparticle-based delivery*

Clinical trials are exploring liposomal formulations of chemotherapeutics like doxorubicin targeting CSCs in ovarian cancer. These formulations enhance drug accumulation at tumor sites.

##### *5.2.1.1.2 Targeted nanocarriers*

Research on functionalized nanoparticles that target CSC markers, such as CD133, is underway, aiming to improve specificity and reduce off-target effects.

##### *5.2.1.1.3 Localized delivery systems*

Injectable hydrogels are being tested for delivering immunotherapeutics directly to tumor sites, improving local drug concentration while minimizing systemic toxicity.

### 5.3 Addressing heterogeneity within tumors

Tumor heterogeneity is a significant challenge in effectively targeting CSCs in gynecological malignancies. This heterogeneity arises from a variety of factors, including genetic mutations, epigenetic modifications, and differential expression of surface markers, resulting in a diverse population of cells within a single tumor. As a result, CSCs can vary not only in their biological properties but also in their responses to therapies, making it difficult to develop universally effective treatment strategies. Understanding and addressing this heterogeneity are crucial for optimizing CSC-targeted therapies and improving clinical outcomes.

To tackle tumor heterogeneity, researchers are exploring multifaceted approaches that combine various therapeutic modalities. For instance, utilizing combination therapies that target multiple pathways simultaneously can help address the adaptive mechanisms employed by CSCs to evade treatment (**Figure 2**). This may involve integrating traditional chemotherapeutic agents with novel targeted therapies or immunotherapies specifically designed to eliminate CSCs. Additionally, personalized medicine approaches, which tailor treatments based on the unique genetic and molecular profile of an individual patient's tumor, hold great promise. By profiling tumors to identify specific mutations and CSC markers, clinicians can select the most appropriate and effective treatment strategies, thereby enhancing the likelihood of achieving meaningful clinical responses.

Furthermore, advances in imaging technologies and single-cell analysis are providing deeper insights into the spatial and temporal dynamics of tumor heterogeneity.

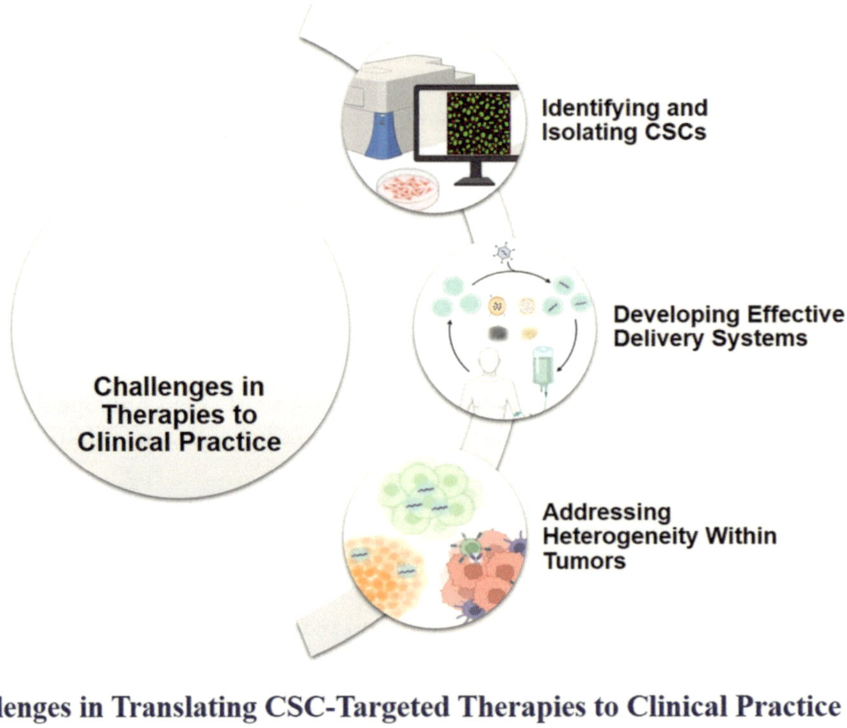


**Figure 2.**
*Challenges in translating cancer stem cell (CSC)-targeted therapies to clinical practice.*

Techniques such as single-cell RNA sequencing allow for the characterization of CSC populations at an unprecedented resolution, revealing insights into their developmental pathways and interactions with the tumor microenvironment. These technologies can guide the identification of novel biomarkers for CSCs and inform the design of therapies that are more likely to target the most aggressive and treatment-resistant cell populations within tumors. By addressing tumor heterogeneity, researchers and clinicians can improve the precision of CSC-targeted therapies, ultimately leading to better treatment outcomes for patients with gynecological cancers [39].

## 6. Future directions in CSC research and therapy

### 6.1 Innovations in targeting CSCs

As research into CSCs progresses, several innovative strategies are emerging to enhance the targeting and eradication of CSCs in gynecological cancers. One promising direction involves the integration of advanced genomic and proteomic technologies that facilitate a deeper understanding of the molecular signatures associated with CSCs. By employing high-throughput sequencing and mass spectrometry, researchers can identify novel biomarkers that distinguish CSCs from non-stem cancer cells, enabling the development of targeted therapies that specifically disrupt CSC pathways. This precision approach not only enhances the likelihood of effective treatment but also minimizes the impact on normal cells, thereby reducing side effects.

Additionally, the application of CRISPR/Cas9 gene-editing technology is poised to revolutionize CSC research. This powerful tool allows for the precise modification of genes associated with CSC maintenance and drug resistance. By selectively knocking out genes that promote CSC properties or overexpressing tumor-suppressive genes, researchers can potentially convert aggressive CSCs into less malignant cell types or make them more susceptible to existing therapies. Furthermore, the development of engineered CAR-T cells specifically designed to target CSC markers represents a cutting-edge strategy in immunotherapy, harnessing the body's immune system to selectively attack and eliminate CSC populations.

Another exciting avenue involves the exploration of the tumor microenvironment (TME) and its role in supporting CSC survival. Emerging research is focusing on how cellular interactions within the TME, such as those with immune cells, fibroblasts, and extracellular matrix components, contribute to CSC characteristics and therapeutic resistance. By developing therapies that disrupt these supportive interactions—either through targeted agents or by reprogramming the immune response—researchers aim to enhance the efficacy of CSC-targeted treatments. As these innovative strategies continue to evolve, they hold the potential to transform the landscape of cancer therapy, leading to more effective and durable treatments for patients with gynecological malignancies [40].

### 6.2 Potential for personalized medicine in gynecological oncology

Personalized medicine is revolutionizing the field of gynecological oncology by tailoring treatment strategies to the individual characteristics of each patient's cancer. This approach relies on understanding the unique genetic, epigenetic, and molecular profiles of a patient's tumor, which can reveal specific vulnerabilities and inform the selection of targeted therapies. For instance, genomic profiling can identify mutations in critical genes associated with drug resistance or aberrant signaling pathways that drive tumor growth. By utilizing this information, clinicians can choose therapies that are more likely to be effective for a particular patient, potentially improving response rates and minimizing unnecessary side effects.

In addition to targeted therapies, personalized medicine in gynecological oncology encompasses immunotherapy and the use of CSC-targeted treatments. By profiling the immune landscape of tumors, clinicians can assess the likelihood of a patient's response to immune checkpoint inhibitors or cancer vaccines. Furthermore, the identification of specific CSC markers allows for the development of therapies designed to selectively eliminate these resistant cell populations. Combining these strategies not only enhances treatment efficacy but also supports the concept of "precision

| **Therapy/approach** | **Mechanism/target** | **Example** | **Clinical trial status** | **Reference** |
|---|---|---|---|---|
| Targeted therapy (monoclonal antibodies) | Targets CSC markers like CD44, ALDH | Anti-CD44 monoclonal antibodies for ovarian cancer | In trials for ovarian cancer (e.g., NCT03091166) | Scott et al. [41] |
| Pathway inhibitors | Inhibits Wnt, Notch, Hedgehog pathways | Wnt inhibitor (LGK974), Notch inhibitor (RO4929097) | Wnt (NCT01351103), Notch (NCT01158158) | Kotipalli et al. [42] |
| Immunotherapy | Enhances immune response against CSCs | Pembrolizumab (PD-1 inhibitor), MUC1 vaccine | NCT02834013 (ovarian cancer), NCT02019524 (MUC1 vaccine) | Patel et al. [43] Kumar et al. [44] |
| CAR-T cells | Genetically engineered T cells targeting CSC markers | CAR-T cells targeting CD44 | In preclinical stages for CSC-specific CAR-T cells | Miller and Maus [45] |
| Nanoparticles | Precision delivery to CSCs via ligand-functionalized particles | Anti-CD44 nanocarriers, PEGylated liposomal doxorubicin | Anti-CD44 nanoparticles in trials for ovarian cancer (NCT01208345) | Garcia and Patel [46] Kumar et al. [47]; Maurya et al. [48] |
| CRISPR/Cas9 gene editing | Gene editing to knock out CSC properties | CRISPR targeting drug-resistant genes in CSCs | Preclinical studies targeting CSC-associated genes | Brown et al. [49] |
| Tumor microenvironment (TME) disruption | Disrupts TME to weaken CSC support | Drugs targeting fibroblasts, immune cells within TME | Ongoing research on CSC and TME interactions in cancer models | Nguyen et al. [50] |
| Personalized medicine | Tailors treatment based on molecular profiles | Genomic and proteomic profiling for individualized therapy | Clinical trials focused on tailored therapies in gynecological cancers | Lee and Wong [51] |
| Artificial intelligence in CSC research | AI-guided analysis of treatment outcomes | AI-based predictive models for personalized therapy selection | Being integrated into clinical decision-making | Johnson et al. [52] |

**Table 1.**
*Overview of current and emerging CSC-targeted therapies in gynecological cancers with clinical trial status.*

oncology," where therapy is tailored not only to the cancer type but also to the individual patient's biological profile.

As the field advances, the integration of artificial intelligence and machine learning is expected to play a pivotal role in personalizing cancer care. These technologies can analyze vast amounts of clinical and genomic data to identify patterns and predict treatment outcomes, guiding clinicians in making more informed decisions. Moreover, ongoing clinical trials focused on personalized approaches will help validate the efficacy of tailored therapies in diverse patient populations. By harnessing the potential of personalized medicine, gynecological oncology is moving toward a future where treatment is not only more effective but also more aligned with the unique biology of each patient's cancer (**Table 1**).

Current therapies targeting CSCs in gynecological cancers focus on several innovative approaches. Targeted therapies using monoclonal antibodies, such as those against CSC markers like CD44 and ALDH, are being explored, particularly in ovarian cancer. Pathway inhibitors that disrupt critical signaling pathways, such as Wnt, Notch, and Hedgehog, are in clinical trials, with examples like LGK974 (Wnt inhibitor) and RO4929097 (Notch inhibitor) showing potential. Immunotherapy, including immune checkpoint inhibitors like pembrolizumab, is being tested in gynecological cancers, with trials such as NCT02834013 for ovarian cancer, alongside the development of CAR-T cells engineered to target CSC-specific markers. Nanotechnology-based therapies are also progressing, with nanoparticles such as anti-CD44 nanocarriers and PEGylated liposomal doxorubicin being trialed for precise CSC targeting and enhanced drug delivery. These novel therapies are undergoing clinical evaluation, aiming to improve treatment efficacy and overcome resistance in gynecological cancers [53].

## 7. Conclusion

This chapter has highlighted the critical role of CSCs in the initiation, progression, and recurrence of gynecological malignancies. CSCs, with their unique capabilities for self-renewal and differentiation, contribute significantly to tumor heterogeneity, metastasis, and resistance to conventional treatments. As a result, they represent a pivotal target in the quest to improve therapeutic outcomes in gynecological cancers.

Advances in understanding the molecular pathways regulating CSC behavior, particularly the Wnt, Notch, and Hedgehog signaling pathways, have opened the door to innovative therapies. Pathway inhibitors, immune-based strategies, and combinatorial treatments are showing promise in preclinical models, with the potential to reduce drug resistance and relapse rates by targeting the root of tumor persistence.

Moreover, integrating CSC-targeted therapies with conventional treatments like chemotherapy and immunotherapy is an exciting development. Such approaches can disrupt the survival mechanisms of CSCs, enhancing treatment efficacy and durability. The future of CSC-targeted strategies will likely align with personalized medicine, tailoring treatments to each patient's unique tumor profile for more precise, effective, and lasting results.

Despite challenges such as CSC heterogeneity and the need for optimized drug delivery systems, the promise of targeting CSCs is transformative. By focusing on eradicating this resilient cell population, oncology is moving closer to achieving more durable and personalized therapies that can significantly improve outcomes for patients with gynecological cancers.

**Author details**

Rama Satya Sri Kotipalli[1*], Mani Sharma[1], Nemala Siva Kumar[2], Abhiram Kumar[3], Chhavi Dhiman[3], Mohini Rawat[4], Piyush Khandelia[3] and Kumar Pranav Narayan[3*]

1 CSIR-Indian Institute of Chemical Technology, Hyderabad, Telangana, India

2 Sri Vasavi Institute of Pharmaceutical Sciences, Pedatadepalli, Andhra Pradesh, India

3 Birla Institute of Technology and Science Pilani, Hyderabad Campus, Hyderabad, Telangana, India

4 Himalayan Institute of Pharmacy and Research, Dehradun, Uttarakhand, India

*Address all correspondence to: satyasri.15247@csiriict.in
and pranav@hyderabad.bits-pilani.ac.in

## References

[1] Eun K, Ham SW, Kim H. Cancer stem cell heterogeneity: Origin and new perspectives on CSC targeting. BMB Reports. 2017;**50**(3):117

[2] Vincent MD. Cancer: Beyond speciation. Advances in Cancer Research. 2011;**112**:283-350

[3] Ramón y Cajal S, Sesé M, Capdevila C, Aasen T, De Mattos-Arruda L, Diaz-Cano SJ, et al. Clinical implications of intratumor heterogeneity: Challenges and opportunities. Journal of Molecular Medicine. 2020;**98**:161-177

[4] Meher JG, Dixit S, Pathan DK, Singh Y, Chandasana H, Pawar VK, et al. Paclitaxel-loaded TPGS enriched self-emulsifying carrier causes apoptosis by modulating survivin expression and inhibits tumour growth in syngeneic mammary tumours. Artificial Cells, Nanomedicine, and Biotechnology. 2018;**46**(Suppl 3):344-358

[5] Aramini B, Masciale V, Arienti C, Dominici M, Stella F, Martinelli G, et al. Cancer stem cells (CSCs), circulating tumor cells (CTCs) and their interplay with cancer associated fibroblasts (CAFs): A new world of targets and treatments. Cancers. 2022;**14**(10):2408

[6] Marzagalli M, Fontana F, Raimondi M, Limonta P. Cancer stem cells—Key players in tumor relapse. Cancers. 2021;**13**(3):376

[7] Papaccio F, Paino F, Regad T, Papaccio G, Desiderio V, Tirino V. Concise review: Cancer cells, cancer stem cells, and mesenchymal stem cells: Influence in cancer development. Stem Cells Translational Medicine. 2017;**6**(12):2115-2125

[8] Sharma M, Ambadipudi SS, Chouhan NK, Nayak VL, Pabbaraja S, Andugulapati SB, et al. Design, synthesis and biological evaluation of novel cationic liposomes loaded with melphalan for the treatment of cancer. Bioorganic & Medicinal Chemistry Letters. 2024;**97**:129549

[9] Shibata M, Hoque MO. Targeting cancer stem cells: A strategy for effective eradication of cancer. Cancers. 2019;**11**(5):732

[10] Mohammed MK, Shao C, Wang J, Wei Q, Wang X, Collier Z, et al. Wnt/β-catenin signaling plays an ever-expanding role in stem cell self-renewal, tumorigenesis and cancer chemoresistance. Genes & Diseases. 2016;**3**(1):11-40

[11] Sharma M, Chouhan NK, Vaidya S, Talati MN. Lipids, peptides, and polymers as targeted drug delivery vectors in cancer therapy. In: Handbook of Research on Advancements in Cancer Therapeutics. IGI Global; 2021. pp. 255-275

[12] Zong X, Nephew KP. Ovarian cancer stem cells: Role in metastasis and opportunity for therapeutic targeting. Cancers. 2019;**11**(7):934

[13] Meisel CT, Porcheri C, Mitsiadis TA. Cancer stem cells, quo vadis? The Notch signaling pathway in tumor initiation and progression. Cells. 2020;**9**(8):1879

[14] Takebe N, Miele L, Harris PJ, Jeong W, Bando H, Kahn M, et al. Targeting Notch, Hedgehog, and Wnt pathways in cancer stem cells: Clinical update. Nature Reviews Clinical Oncology. 2015;**12**(8):445-464

[15] Agliano A, Calvo A, Box C. The challenge of targeting cancer stem cells

to halt metastasis. Seminars in Cancer Biology. 2017;**44**:25-42. DOI: 10.1016/j.semcancer.2017.03.003. Epub 2017 Mar 18

[16] Arcaroli JJ, Dasari A, Messersmith WA, Jimeno A. γ-Secretase inhibitors in solid tumor malignancies. Drugs of the Future. 2011;**36**(9):677

[17] Sabol M, Trnski D, Musani V, Ozretić P, Levanat S. Role of GLI transcription factors in pathogenesis and their potential as new therapeutic targets. International Journal of Molecular Sciences. 2018;**19**(9):2562

[18] Cochrane CR, Szczepny A, Watkins DN, Cain JE. Hedgehog signaling in the maintenance of cancer stem cells. Cancers. 2015;**7**(3):1554-1585

[19] Justilien V, Fields AP. Molecular pathways: Novel approaches for improved therapeutic targeting of hedgehog signaling in cancer stem cells. Clinical Cancer Research. 2015;**21**(3):505-513

[20] Wang Q, Peng H, Qi X, Wu M, Zhao X. Targeted therapies in gynecological cancers: A comprehensive review of clinical evidence. Signal Transduction and Targeted Therapy. 2020;**5**(1):137

[21] Marquardt S, Solanki M, Spitschak A, Vera J, Puetzer BM. Emerging functional markers for cancer stem cell-based therapies: Understanding signaling networks for targeting metastasis. Seminars in Cancer Biology. 2018;**53**:90-109. DOI: 10.1016/j.semcancer.2018.06.006. Epub 2018 Jun 30

[22] Hass R, von der Ohe J, Ungefroren H. Impact of the tumor microenvironment on tumor heterogeneity and consequences for cancer cell plasticity and stemness. Cancers. 2020;**12**(12):3716

[23] Kharkar PS. Cancer stem cell (CSC) inhibitors in oncology—A promise for a better therapeutic outcome: State of the art and future perspectives. Journal of Medicinal Chemistry. 2020;**63**(24):15279-15307

[24] Akbarzadeh M, Akbarzadeh S, Majidinia M. Targeting notch signaling pathway as an effective strategy in overcoming drug resistance in ovarian cancer. Pathology, Research and Practice. 2020;**216**(11):153158

[25] Aguilar-Gallardo C, Rutledge EC, Martínez-Arroyo AM, Hidalgo JJ, Domingo S, Simón C. Overcoming challenges of ovarian cancer stem cells: Novel therapeutic approaches. Stem Cell Reviews and Reports. 2012;**8**:994-1010

[26] Borlongan MC, Wang H. Profiling and targeting cancer stem cell signaling pathways for cancer therapeutics. Frontiers in Cell and Developmental Biology. 2023;**11**:1125174

[27] Zhang D, Tang DG, Rycaj K. Cancer stem cells: Regulation programs, immunological properties and immunotherapy. Seminars in Cancer Biology. 2018;**52**(Pt 2):94-106. DOI: 10.1016/j.semcancer.2018.05.001. Epub 2018 May 9

[28] Ruiu R, Tarone L, Rolih V, Barutello G, Bolli E, Riccardo F, et al. Cancer stem cell immunology and immunotherapy: Harnessing the immune system against cancer's source. Progress in Molecular Biology and Translational Science. 2019;**164**:119-188

[29] Garg P, Ramisetty SK, Subbalakshmi AR, Krishna M, Pareek S, Mohanty A, et al. Gynecological cancer tumor microenvironment: Unveiling cellular complexity and therapeutic potential. Biochemical Pharmacology. 2024;**229**:116498

[30] De Francesco EM, Sotgia F, Lisanti MP. Cancer stem cells (CSCs): Metabolic strategies for their identification and eradication. Biochemical Journal. 2018;**475**(9):1611-1634

[31] Keyvani V, Riahi E, Yousefi M, Esmaeili SA, Shafabakhsh R, Moradi Hasan-Abad A, et al. Gynecologic cancer, cancer stem cells, and possible targeted therapies. Frontiers in Pharmacology. 2022;**13**:823572

[32] Diamandis M, White NM, Yousef GM. Personalized medicine: Marking a new epoch in cancer patient management. Molecular Cancer Research. 2010;**8**(9):1175-1187

[33] Sharma M, Kotipalli RSS, Kumar NS, Kumar A, Rawat M, Dhiman C, Kumar M. Innovations in Drug Delivery Strategies for Breast Cancer. IntechOpen; 2024

[34] Sistigu A, Musella M, Galassi C, Vitale I, De Maria R. Tuning cancer fate: Tumor microenvironment's role in cancer stem cell quiescence and reawakening. Frontiers in Immunology. 2020;**11**:2166

[35] Spencer DA, Auffinger BM, Murphy JP, Muroski EM, Qiao J, Gorind Y, et al. Hitting a moving target: Glioma stem cells demand new approaches in glioblastoma therapy. Current Cancer Drug Targets. 2017;**17**(3):236-254

[36] Zubor P, Dankova Z, Kolkova Z, Holubekova V, Brany D, Mersakova S, et al. Rho GTPases in gynecologic cancers: In-depth analysis toward the paradigm change from reactive to predictive, preventive, and personalized medical approach benefiting the patient and healthcare. Cancers. 2020;**12**(5):1292

[37] Muralikrishnan V, Hurley TD, Nephew KP. Targeting aldehyde dehydrogenases to eliminate cancer stem cells in gynecologic malignancies. Cancers. 2020;**12**(4):961

[38] Sharma M, Joshi J, Chouhan NK, Talati MN, Vaidya S, Kumar A. Liposome-A comprehensive approach for researchers. In: Molecular Pharmacology. IntechOpen; 2020

[39] Das S, Das MK, Chakraborty T. Cancer stem cell targeting for anticancer therapy: Strategies and challenges. In: Topics in Anti-Cancer Research. Vol. 8. Bentham Science Publisher; 2019. pp. 97-156. DOI: 10.2174/9789811404382119080007

[40] Sharma M, Kansal S. A comprehensive study of multi-drug resistance in tuberculosis: Help desk for researchers, doctors, and patients. In: Contemporary Issues in Global Medicine and Moving Toward International Healthcare Equity. IGI Global; 2022. pp. 317-347

[41] Scott EC, Baines AC, Gong Y, Moore R Jr, Pamuk GE, Saber H, et al. Trends in the approval of cancer therapies by the FDA in the twenty-first century. Nature Reviews Drug Discovery. 2023;**22**(8):625-640

[42] Kotipalli RSS, Patnaik SS, Kumar JM, Ramakrishna S, Muralidharan K. Biochanin-A attenuates DHEA-induced polycystic ovary syndrome via upregulation of GDF9 and BMP15 signaling in vivo. Life Sciences. 2023;**326**:121795

[43] Patel DM, Mateen R, Qaddour N, Carrillo A, Verschraegen C, Yang Y, et al. A comprehensive review of immunotherapy clinical trials for metastatic urothelial carcinoma: Immune checkpoint inhibitors alone or in combination, novel antibodies, cellular therapies, and vaccines. Cancers. 2024;**16**(2):335

[44] Kumar A, Sakhare K, Bhattacharya D, Chattopadhyay R, Parikh P, Narayan KP, et al. Communication in non-communicable diseases (NCDs) and role of immunomodulatory nutraceuticals in their management. Frontiers in Nutrition. 2022;**9**:966152

[45] Miller BC, Maus MV. CD19-targeted CAR T cells: A new tool in the fight against B cell malignancies. Oncology Research and Treatment. 2015;**38**(12):683-690

[46] Patnaik SS, Kotipalli R, Jerald MK, Muralidharan K. Combination treatment of recombinant growth differentiation factor-9 and Cetrorelix improves gestational origin of the polycystic ovarian syndrome in female rats. Life Sciences. 2023;**321**:121638. DOI: 10.1016/j.lfs.2023.121638. Epub 2023 Mar 29

[47] Kumar A, Rana R, Saklani R, Kumar M, Yadav PK, Tiwari A, et al. Technology transfer of a validated RP-HPLC method for the simultaneous estimation of andrographolide and paclitaxel in application to pharmaceutical nanoformulation. Journal of Chromatographic Science. 2024;**62**(4):356-363

[48] Maurya P, Saklani R, Singh S, Nisha R, Mishra N, Singh P, et al. Effective uptake of folate-functionalized ethionamide-loaded hybrid system: Targeting alveolar macrophages. Nanomedicine. 2022;**17**(24):1819-1831

[49] Brown EA, Eikenbary SR, Landis WG. Bayesian network-based risk assessment of synthetic biology: Simulating CRISPR-Cas9 gene drive dynamics in invasive rodent management. Risk Analysis. 2022;**42**(12):2835-2846

[50] Nguyen TM, Ngoc DTM, Choi JH, Lee CH. Unveiling the neural environment in cancer: Exploring the role of neural circuit players and potential therapeutic strategies. Cells. 2023;**12**(15):1996

[51] Syn NL, Yong WP, Goh BC, Lee SC. Evolving landscape of tumor molecular profiling for personalized cancer therapy: A comprehensive review. Expert Opinion on Drug Metabolism & Toxicology. 2016;**12**(8):911-922

[52] Johnson KB, Wei WQ, Weeraratne D, Frisse ME, Misulis K, Rhee K, et al. Precision medicine, AI, and the future of personalized health care. Clinical and Translational Science. 2021;**14**(1):86-93

[53] Dianat-Moghadam H, Heidarifard M, Jahanban-Esfahlan R, Panahi Y, Hamishehkar H, Pouremamali F, et al. Cancer stem cells-emanated therapy resistance: Implications for liposomal drug delivery systems. Journal of Controlled Release. 2018;**288**:62-83